Minimal Incision Surgery

Editor

NEAL M. BLITZ

CLINICS IN PODIATRIC MEDICINE AND SURGERY

www.podiatric.theclinics.com

Consulting Editor
THOMAS J. CHANG

January 2025 • Volume 42 • Number 1

ELSEVIER

1600 John F. Kennedy Boulevard • Suite 1800 • Philadelphia, Pennsylvania, 19103-2899

http://www.theclinics.com

CLINICS IN PODIATRIC MEDICINE AND SURGERY Volume 42, Number 1
January 2025 ISSN 0891-8422, ISBN-13: 978-0-443-29360-3

Editor: Megan Ashdown
Developmental Editor: Anita Chamoli

Clinics in Podiatric Medicine and Surgery (ISSN 0891-8422) is published quarterly by Elsevier Inc., 360 Park Avenue South, New York, NY 10010-1710. Months of issue are January, April, July, and October. Business and Editorial Offices: 1600 John F. Kennedy Blvd., Ste. 1800, Philadelphia, PA 19103-2899. Customer Service Office: 3251 Riverport Lane, Maryland Heights, MO 63043. Periodicals postage paid at New York, NY and additional mailing offices. Subscription prices are $336.00 per year for US individuals, $100.00 per year for US students and residents, $422.00 per year for Canadian individuals, $510.00 for international individuals, $100.00 per year for Canadian students/residents, and $220.00 per year for foreign students/residents. For institutional access pricing please contact Customer Service via the contact information below. To receive student/resident rate, orders must be accompanied by name of affiliated institution, date of term, and the *signature* of program/residency coordinator on institution letterhead. Orders will be billed at individual rate until proof of status is received. Foreign air speed delivery is included in all *Clinics* subscription prices. All prices are subject to change without notice. Orders, claims, and journal inquiries: Please visit our Support Hub page https://service.elsevier.com for assistance.

Reprints. For copies of 100 or more of articles in this publication, please contact the Commercial Reprints Department, Elsevier Inc., 360 Park Avenue South, New York, NY 10010-1710. Tel.: 212-633-3874; Fax: 212-633-3820; E-mail: reprints@elsevier.com.

Clinics in Podiatric Medicine and Surgery is covered in *MEDLINE/PubMed (Index Medicus) and EMBASE/Excerpta Medica.*

Contributors

CONSULTING EDITOR

THOMAS J. CHANG, DPM
Clinical Professor and Past Chairman, Department of Podiatric Surgery, California College of Podiatric Medicine Faculty, The Podiatry Institute, Santa Rosa, California, USA

EDITOR

NEAL M. BLITZ, DPM, FACFAS
Private Practice, Blitz Footcare, New York, New York, USA; Private Practice, Blitz Footcare, Beverly Hills, California, USA

AUTHORS

NEAL M. BLITZ, DPM, FACFAS
Private Practice, Blitz Footcare, New York, New York, USA; Private Practice, Blitz Footcare, Beverly Hills, California, USA

ERIC S. BASKIN, DPM, FACFAS
Private Practitioner, Advocare Stafford Orthopedics, Manahawkin, New Jersey, USA

TIAGO BAUMFELD, MD, PhD
Foot and Ankle Surgeon, Foot and Ankle Unit, Hospital Felício Rocho, Belo Horizonte, Minas Gerais, Brazil

FELIPE CHAPARRO RAVAZZANO, MD
Medical Surgeon, Department of Orthopedic Surgery, Foot and Ankle Center, Clínica Universidad de los Andes, Chile

DHAVEL D. CHAUHAN, DPM, AACFAS
Fellow, Dallas Advanced Foot and Ankle Reconstruction Fellowship, Dallas, Texas, USA

LEIF CLAASSEN, MD
Physician, Department of Trauma, Hand and Reconstructive Surgery, Jena University Hospital, Jena, Germany

KRIS A. DI NUCCI, DPM, FACFAS
Podiatric Foot and Ankle Surgeon, Private Practice, Foot and Ankle Center of Arizona, Scottsdale, Arizona, USA

DAVID GORDON, MB ChB, MRCS, MD, FRCS (Tr & Orth)
Consultant Orthopaedic Foot and Ankle Surgeon, The London Clinic, London, United Kingdom

BOGDAN GRECEA, DPM, AACFAS
Clinical Assistant Professor, Department of Podiatric Medicine & Surgery, Western University of Health Science, New York, New York, USA; Department of Foot and Ankle Surgery, Blitz Footcare, Penthouse, Beverly Hills, California, USA

MATTHEW GREENBLATT, DPM, AACFAS
Fellowship Trained Foot and Ankle Surgeon, International Center of Limb Lengthening, Rubin Institute of Advanced Orthopedics, Baltimore, Maryland, USA

KAJETAN KLOS, MD
Physician, Department of Orthopedics and Traumatology, University Medical Center of the Johannes Gutenberg University, Mainz, Germany

TOGAY KOÇ, MBBS, MSc, FRCS (Tr & Orth)
Consultant, University Hospital Southampton NHS Foundation Trust, Southampton, United Kingdom

THOMAS L. LEWIS, MBChB (Hons), BSc (Hons), FRCS (Tr & Orth), MFSTEd
Trauma and Orthopaedic Specialty ST8 Registrar, King's College Hospital NHS Foundation NHS Trust, London, United Kingdom

BRIAN G. LODER, DPM, FACFAS
Fellowship Director, Michigan Minimal invasive and Reconstructive Foot and Ankle Fellowship, Clinton Township, Michigan, USA

SARA MATEEN, DPM, AACFAS
Fellowship Trained Foot and Ankle Surgeon, International Center of Limb Lengthening, Rubin Institute of Advanced Orthopedics, Baltimore, Maryland, USA

NEHAL MODHA, DPM, AACFAS
Podiatric Surgeon, McKinney Footcare, Mckinney, Texas, USA

GUSTAVO ARAUJO NUNES, MD, PhD(C)
Foot and Ankle Surgeon, Foot and Ankle Unit, COTE Brasília Clinic, Federal District, Brazil

ADAM REANEY, BSc (Hons), MRCPod, LLCM, ARSM
Podiatrist and Medical Student, Cardiff University School of Medicine, Cardiff, United Kingdom

DAVID REDFERN, MD
Consultant Trauma Orthopaedic Surgeon, Cleveland Clinic London, London, United Kingdom; Montefiore Hospital, Hove, East Sussex, England

KLAUS EDGAR ROTH, MD
Physician, Department of Orthopedic Surgery, Gelenkzentrum Rheinmain, Hochheim, Germany

CALVIN J. RUSHING, DPM, FACFAS
Board Certified, Fellowship-Trained, Podiatric Surgeon, Director, Dallas Advanced Foot and Ankle Reconstruction Fellowship, Dallas Orthopedic and Shoulder Institute, Sunnyvale, Texas, USA

FRANCISCO SÁNCHEZ VILLANUEVA, MD
Department of Orthopedic Surgery, Foot and Ankle Center, Clínica Puerto Varas y Puerto Montt, Chile

NOMAN A. SIDDIQUI, DPM, MHA, FACFAS
Attending Physician, Division of Orthopedic Surgery, Hackensack Meridian Health, Hackensack, New Jersey, USA; Division of Podiatric Surgery, Sinai Hospital, Baltimore, Maryland, USA

JOEL VERNOIS, MD
Trauma and Orthopaedic Surgeon, ICP, Clinique Blomet, Paris, France; Sussex Orthopaedic NHS Treatment Centre, Haywards Heath, England

HAZIBULLAH WAIZY, MD
Surgeon, Department of Orthopedics, Orthoprofis, Hannover, Germany

DAVID T. WONG, DPM, FACFAS
Director of Foot Surgery, Department of Orthopedics, BronxCare Health System, Bronx, New York, USA

Contents

> The journey through the history of minimally invasive surgery in foot and ankle procedures reveals a remarkable narrative of innovation and progress. Minimally invasive surgery has been adopted in various foot and ankle procedures including elective and trauma surgery. Most notably, the transformative impact of minimally invasive bunion surgery, spanning now 6 generation techniques, showcases a relentless pursuit of precision and efficiency. The incorporation of beveled screws in the latest generation stands as a testament to the ongoing biomechanical and research-driven advancements that contribute to the ultimate stability and success of minimally invasive procedures.

> The revival of "new" minimally invasive bunion surgery (MIBS) is made possible as a laparoscopic-like fluoroscopically guided procedure using new instrumentation, advanced osseous realignment techniques and procedure-specific orthopedic hardware. Bunions of all severities can be treated with MIBS with a functional walking recovery in a small surgical shoe. Realignment occurs through a subcapital osteotomy with metatarsal head shifts that are stabilized by a single or dual metatarsal MIBS screw(s) that span a resultant osseous defect. Bone healing occurs by callus deposition, a process of "first metatarsal regeneration," resulting in a new straight realigned first metatarsal segment. New MIBS is rapidly evolving with widespread use and we are currently on the fifth & sixth generational update, highlighting a 1-screw construct. Surgeons are rapidly flocking to learn and incorporate this modern procedure in their daily practice.

> Hammer toe deformity is a highly prevalent lesser toe deformity and accounts for a high proportion of appointments to foot and ankle clinics. Its etiology is due to extrinsic and intrinsic muscular imbalance, attenuation and subsequent rupture of the plantar plate, and neuromuscular disorders. This leads to marked flexion of the proximal interphalangeal joint and extension of the metatarsophalangeal joint. Effective diagnosis requires robust clinical examination and radiographic imaging or MRI. This

article discusses the anatomy, etiology, and management of hammer toe deformity using percutaneous surgical techniques, as well as a treatment algorithm.

Eric S. Baskin

Complex forefoot deformities are challenging to treat and are labor intensive for the surgeon and the patient. New minimally invasive surgery (MIS) shows great potential and in some instances outperforms traditional open surgery. Another advantage MIS has is that it is technically easier to perform (once proficient) and produces less pain and recovery for the patient. This article takes the reader through MIS preoperative planning, soft tissue considerations, the different osteotomy configuration options, rationale, transverse plane correction, sagittal plane correction, revision MIS surgery of malunions, metatarsus adductus correction, hybrid MIS correction, and postoperative bandaging and management.

Joel Vernois, David Redfern, and Eric S. Baskin

Lapidus is a common procedure in our armamentarium for the treatment of hallux valgus deformity. This study presents to the reader that it can be performed percutaneously. It is a technically difficult procedure to perform that requires didactic and cadaveric percutaneous training.

Klaus Edgar Roth, Kajetan Klos, Leif Claassen, and Hazibullah Waizy

A variety of osteotomies on the calcaneus have been described in the past to adapt the shape of the calcaneus to specific needs. Newer osteotomy and fixation methods allow the procedure to be as minimally invasive as possible. Recent data suggest that the minimally invasive surgery (MIS) techniques allow for fewer complications, particularly with regard to wound healing. The calcaneus can be cut and shifted in all planes, shortened, and rotated with MIS. Calcaneal MIS has become a major component of foot and ankle surgery.

Brian G. Loder

This article will discuss the risk and benefits of percutaneous arthrodesis of various joints in the foot. This will focus on the surgical indications, the approach, as well as tips and pearls to enhance the outcomes of the procedures. Lastly, it will discuss post-surgical protocol and the postoperative complications that are particular to the percutaneous approach.

David T. Wong

Hallux valgus recurrence after traditional open bunion surgery is a notable concern. New minimally invasive bunion surgery (MIBS) offers a promising new revision option for those with recurrent hallux valgus. This innovative approach signifies a noteworthy departure from traditional open surgical methods by minimizing tissue damage, allowing immediate weight bearing, and providing improved patient satisfaction outcomes. This article provides is insights into this emerging method, case examples, and key surgical treatment pearls for treating the recurrent bunion with MIBS. As more surgeons gain MIBS experience, this approach will likely become the gold standard revision method for revisions.

Over the last 5 years, minimally invasive surgery (MIS) has seen a significant surge, propelled by advancements in surgical equipment, implants, methodologies, and comprehensive education. The introduction of specialized hardware and advanced bone-cutting burrs has contributed to a reduction in complications. Evidence from peer-reviewed studies suggests that the outcomes of MIS are often on par with, and at times surpass, those of traditional surgical methods. In the context of MIS, certain complications are specifically linked to the use of burrs and hardware, the types of deformities being addressed, and the tools utilized. This article aims to discuss these complications associated with MIS.

Minimally invasive surgery is gaining tremendous popularity in reconstructive foot and ankle surgery, as well as with trauma. Minimally invasive approaches have demonstrated equivalent to outcomes to traditional open incisional approaches with the added benefit of less risk for wound healing complications and surgical site infections. Advances in orthopedic hardware and surgical techniques are allowing minimal incision surgery for trauma to become more widespread. While there is a steeper learning curve to become proficient, minimally invasive surgery is likely to become the standard for most foot and ankle trauma cases.

New minimally invasive bunion surgery for hallux valgus (HV) has received attention in the last few years. A rapid growth in knowledge and techniques has been seen, with many publications, books, and experienced surgeons worldwide. Several variational advancements have emerged with the most common as a percutaneous subcapital osteotomy first metatarsal with long scaffolding minimally invasive (MI) screw placement. MI techniques are a great advancement in the treatment of all HV severities. Supportive literature has demonstrated that MI can achieve equal to better results compared to traditional open surgery, for metrics such as satisfaction, pain, and time to full recovery.

Minimally invasive surgery (MIS) continues to develop as a viable alternative to traditional open surgery for various foot and ankle pathologies. The neuropathic foot is one area where MIS can be very beneficial to surgeons and their patients. Improving wound healing and decreasing the surgical footprint and thus reducing complications associated with soft tissue in this population is advantageous. Further research is necessary; however, the early successful outcomes in neuroarthropathy reconstruction via MIS are encouraging.

CLINICS IN PODIATRIC MEDICINE AND SURGERY

THE CLINICS ARE AVAILABLE ONLINE!
Access your subscription at:
www.theclinics.com

Foreword

Minimal Incision Surgery

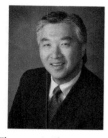

Thomas J. Chang, DPM
Consulting Editor

I remember the Minimal Incision Surgery (MIS) movement in the 1970s to 1980s. Back then, MIS was often the first opportunity for surgeons to try their hand at foot surgery and often resulted in poor outcomes. Some of them were completely disastrous, with irreversible damage to the neurovascular and osseous tissues within the foot. Many osteotomies were left unfixated, and forefoot complications were commonly seen.

This new movement of MIS has a new philosophy and perspective. Many of the current pioneers are talented "open" surgeons who have excellent knowledge of surgical procedures and principles. Simply stated, surgeons are now just performing existing surgical procedures through smaller and smaller incisions and have studied their techniques and outcomes closely. MIS is slowly evolving into a science and not just a fad of the past.

It is exciting to present this current update on "Minimal Incision Surgery." There has been a tremendous resurgence of interest over the past 5 years, and it is an area of enthusiasm not only within the United States, but equally seen around the world. This is an extremely timely issue and one I hope you will review with an open mind.

As with any new innovation, please take the time to train properly and thoroughly. There are many opportunities for first-time training, and repeated training is recommended. Take it seriously, and your patients will truly be the ones who benefit from your commitment.

I applaud Dr Neal Blitz and his MIS colleagues in sharing their skills and knowledge within this issue. The topics range from forefoot surgery, with an expected concentration on MIS bunion surgery, to many other areas of the foot to include Charcot

Clin Podiatr Med Surg 42 (2025) xiii–xiv
https://doi.org/10.1016/j.cpm.2024.10.002
0891-8422/25/© 2024 Published by Elsevier Inc.

deformities. It is an interesting time for the foot and ankle surgeon as this movement continues to grow. I know I will be watching…

Thomas J. Chang, DPM
Sonoma County Orthopedic/Podiatric Specialists
3536 Mendocino Avenue, Suite 300B
Santa Rosa, CA 95403, USA

E-mail address:
thomaschang14@comcast.net

Preface

Minimally Invasive Surgery: Ignore It Until You Can't

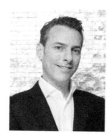

Neal M. Blitz, DPM
Editor

Change is difficult, especially when it comes to our surgical skill set. Many of us have spent years mastering our craft, fine-tuning the hand-eye coordination and muscle memory required to consistently deliver successful outcomes for our patients. As a result, the threshold for adopting new techniques must be high. Yet, in recent years, minimally invasive surgery (MIS) has rapidly gained momentum, pushing surgeons to consider whether they should integrate these procedures into their practices.

The resurgence of MIS is largely credited to advancements in surgical instrumentation, the development of specialized orthopedic implants, and refined techniques that are producing consistently positive patient outcomes. However, adopting these procedures is no small feat—it requires learning a completely new set of skills that are difficult to master, as well as rethinking how many conditions are treated and managed. As such, there is significant resistance among surgeons to abandon trusted, time-tested practices.

A large portion of surgeons remain skeptical, particularly in a profession that has traditionally been fusion-focused. Many take a cautious observer's stance, waiting for robust, supportive literature before even considering these techniques. Even early adopters tend to "dip a toe in the water," opting for a gradual, "see it to believe it" approach to determine if MIS truly has staying power.

But today, MIS seems to have reached a critical threshold. This is no longer a fleeting trend; MIS is here to stay and will continue to evolve in the coming years. As the body of evidence grows and the advantages become undeniable, even the surgeons who were once hesitant are now rushing to gain training and hands-on experience. If MIS were easy to perform, it would have already overtaken traditional surgical practices. The fact that it hasn't underscores the challenges involved in mastering this approach.

Clin Podiatr Med Surg 42 (2025) xv–xvi
https://doi.org/10.1016/j.cpm.2024.10.001
0891-8422/25/© 2024 Published by Elsevier Inc.

The real question for surgeons isn't "if not now, when?" but rather "if not now, how?" How can we successfully adopt these techniques and gain the necessary expertise to ensure the same level of patient safety and outcomes we have spent years perfecting with traditional methods?

The truth is the future of surgery will likely involve an increasing reliance on minimally invasive techniques. The profession is at a crossroads. Surgeons who choose to ignore the evolution of MIS may soon find themselves on the sidelines of a rapidly changing field. For those willing to embrace this new challenge, the rewards are likely to be great—not just for their own professional development, but more importantly, for the well-being of their patients.

Neal M. Blitz, DPM
Private Practice, Blitz Footcare
800A 5th Avenue, Suite 403
New York, NY 10065, USA

435 North Roxbury Drive, Penthouse
Beverly Hills, CA 90210, USA

E-mail address:
drblitz@drnealblitz.com

The History and Instrumentation of Minimally Invasive Pedal Surgery

Bogdan Grecea, DPM, AACFAS[a,b,*]

KEYWORDS

- Minimally invasive surgery • Minimally invasive bunion surgery • Chamfered screw
- Rotary bur

KEY POINTS

- Minimally invasive surgery (MIS) transformed traditional procedures through smaller incisions and quicker recoveries.
- Discoveries of x-ray and fluoroscopy revolutionized diagnostics and guided surgeries, significantly shaping minimally invasive techniques.
- The low-speed high torque rotary bur is ideal for controlled osteotomies.
- Adoption of atraumatic techniques that MIS provides prioritizes gentle tissue handling to preserve blood supply and minimize soft tissue damage—aligning with improved patient outcomes.
- MIS is used for a wide variety of elective (bunion, hammertoe, reconstructive) and nonelective (trauma) surgeries.

INTRODUCTION

Over the course of medical history, the evolution of surgical techniques has been marked by transformative milestones that have not only redefined patient care but also reshaped the landscape of modern medicine. Among these groundbreaking advancements is the advent of minimally invasive surgery (MIS), which stands out as a revolutionary chapter in surgical practice across all medical specialties. This innovative approach is characterized by smaller incisions, reduced tissue trauma, and faster recovery times. Not only has MIS elevated patient outcomes but has fundamentally transformed the traditional surgical treatment paradigm of many conditions in the foot and ankle.

[a] Department of Foot and Ankle Surgery, Blitz Footcare, 800A 5th Avenue, Suite 403, New York, NY 10065, USA; [b] Department of Foot and Ankle Surgery, Blitz Footcare, 435 N. Roxbury Dr., Penthouse, Beverly Hills, CA 90210, USA
* Department of Foot and Ankle Surgery, Blitz Footcare, 800A 5th Avenue, Suite 403, New York, NY 10065.
E-mail address: bgrecea@gmail.com

Clin Podiatr Med Surg 42 (2025) 1–9
https://doi.org/10.1016/j.cpm.2024.09.005
0891-8422/25/© 2024 Elsevier Inc. All rights are reserved, including those for text and data mining, AI training, and similar technologies.

podiatric.theclinics.com

Minimally invasive did not simply come into existence overnight but rather a slow journey of continual additive medical advancements over time. The origins span several medical and surgical specialties. Innovations, in some cases, began as "early experiments" that evolved into the sophistication of present day MIS. Minimally invasive pedal surgery is made possible through the advent of laparoscopic surgery, fluoroscopy, rotary burs, and innovative medical implants.

THE LAPAROSCOPY SPARK

The groundwork/foundation for the development of the laparoscope started in 1805 with an early version of endoscope called the Lichtleiter (light conductor) by Philip Bozzini used to examine the interior of the human body. Several iterations and developments throughout the years allowed for the first laparoscopic surgery to be performed in dogs in 1901 and subsequently in 1910 in humans with rudimentary instruments compared with contemporary versions.[1,2] The field of general surgery was transformed through the development and introduction of fiber optic cables and miniature video cameras in the 1960s and 1980s, respectively, which allowed for better illumination and visualization of internal organs while viewing the surgical field on a video monitor. Dr Kurt Semm, a German gynecologist, performed the first laparoscopic appendectomy in 1981.[3] This was met with immediate skepticism and the German Surgical Society suggested he be suspended from medical practice. He attempted to publish his work and was rejected on grounds of "unethical" technique.[4,5] He is now considered the father of modern laparoscopic surgery as he demonstrated the practical applications of laparoscopic techniques in general surgery, and this has become the gold standard.

Laparoscopy's success and widespread adoption significantly influenced the development of MIS across various medical specialties, including orthopedics and podiatry. The principles of reducing surgical trauma, minimizing recovery times, and improving patient outcomes became guiding tenets for other fields of medicine.

IMPACT OF FLUOROSCOPY

Similar to how laparoscopic surgery transformed general surgery, the advent of fluoroscopy allowed orthopedic conditions to be treated through smaller incisions. Fluoroscopy is a form of medical imagining that provides continuous x-ray images on a monitor in a movie-like fashion. Fluoroscopy began with the discovery of x-rays by Wilhelm Conrad Roentgen in 1895.[6–8] One year later, Thomas Edison developed the first "fluoroscope" which consisted of a fluorescent screen and an x-ray source, allowing real-time viewing of the body's internal structures. The fluoroscope was flawed as it resulted in high levels of x-ray radiation. Both Edison and his assistant Clarence Dally were exposed to large doses of radiation, resulting in the death of Dally due to cancer and the cessation of fluoroscope investigations by Edison.

It was not until the 1950s that the advent of the image intensifier reduced the radiation exposure and significantly improved the clarity of the images. The image intensifier converts x-rays into a more visible light that allows for viewing on a monitor. Throughout the 1980s and 1990s, the digital technology revolution allowed the traditional photographic film to be replaced allowing for even lower doses of radiation, better image storage, and retrieval capabilities. Today, extremity-specific fluoroscopic mobile units allow for high resolution images minimizing radiation to the operator. The units have a C-arm swivel that allows anteroposterior and lateral images with ease and simplicity, necessary for proper visualization with MIS techniques (**Fig. 1**).

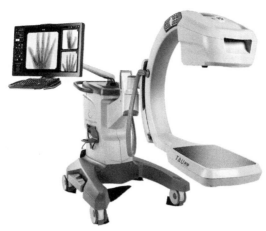

Fig. 1. Example of a mini fluoroscopy unit allowing for high resolution images while minimizing radiation. The unit has a swivel that allows for intraoperative anteroposterior and lateral images. Pictured is an Orthoscan mobile mini C-arm. (*With permission from* Orthoscan Inc, Scottsdale, AZ.)

Additionally, the extremity units are capable of a single operator without the need for radiology professionals to work and move the unit.

THE LOW SPEED HIGH TORQUE BUR AND CONSOLE SYSTEM

The high speed-low torque console system is widely utilized throughout foot and ankle surgery, and most of us are very familiar with these systems as they are the mainstay for traditional/open procedures. This system is often used in procedures requiring rapid cutting (sawing systems) or ablation of tissues where precision is essential. The revolutions per minute (RPMs) range into the tens of thousands.

Conversely, MIS uses console systems with low speed high torque (LSHT) (**Fig. 2**). This was developed to reduce soft tissue trauma by operating at lower speeds/RPMs to minimize heat generation and vibration to prevent skin and bone thermal necrosis. This system also offers the surgeon intuitive control over the bur's settings/parameters such as speed, torque, and irrigation flow based on specific requirements. The RPMs range into the hundreds to thousands, making it the ideal system for MIS.

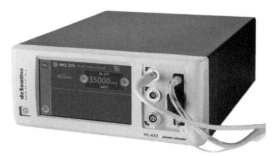

Fig. 2. Example of LSHT console system used for MIS. (*From* Pictured is a De Soutter Medical PC-472 Power Console, De Soutter Medical Limited, United Kingdom.)

THE SURGICAL ROTARY BUR

The creation of the first surgical bur for dental procedures is often attributed to Dr John Borden and Dr William H. Morrison.[9] In the 1950s, they collaborated to develop the air-driven, high-speed handpiece for dental drills. This innovation marked a significant advancement in dental technology, allowing for more efficient and precise tooth preparation during various dental procedures. The design of the surgical bur allowed for a rotary motion, making it well-suited for tasks that required precise cutting. The success and effectiveness of the surgical bur in dentistry eventually led to its adoption in various medical fields, including general surgery and orthopedics. The versatility and precision of the surgical bur made it a valuable tool for a wide range of surgical procedures beyond its initial dental applications.

Upon initial adaptation of the surgical bur into other fields, it was used mainly in destructive fashion, for the denuding of joint cartilage or removing exostoses, given the shape of the bur ("pineapple," "christmas tree"). However, as the field advanced, so did the bur design. During the late 20th century, significant advancements in minimally invasive surgical techniques spurred the development of various types/designs of surgical burs, as seen in **Fig. 3**, each serving a different purpose/intent.

The most relevant bur design for foot and ankle surgery was made by Dr Alan Shannon, for precise bone cutting and shaping. An example of this bur is seen in **Fig. 4**, along with its anatomy. The active portion of the bur encompassess the bur tip and body, which serve different purposes. The bur tip is sharp and used for penetrating dense cortical bone. The body of the bur is often used in a seesaw motion to cut spongy cancellous bone. The smooth/inactive portion of the bur is highly important as this can be laid against skin or soft tissue without engagement which serves as protection when paired with irrigation.

THE DRIVING FORCE

As a general concept for both elective and trauma surgery, the first basic tenet of AO principles is: "Atraumatic Technique: Handle tissues gently and with care, preserving blood supply, and minimizing soft tissue damage during surgery."[10] This principle underscores the importance of minimizing trauma to the surrounding tissues during surgical procedures. By adopting atraumatic techniques, surgeons aim to preserve the blood supply, reduce inflammation, and promote faster healing. This approach aligns with the overall goal of achieving successful surgical alignment/correction while minimizing additional damage to the patient's surrounding tissues which remain untouched.

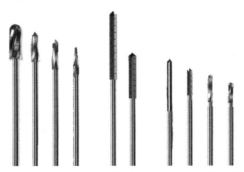

Fig. 3. Example of various types of minimally invasive burs with different shapes serving different purposes. (*With permission from* Percutaneous Burs, Orthocape.)

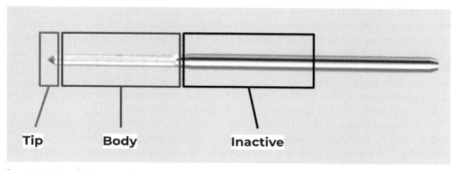

Tip   **Body**   **Inactive**

Fig. 4. Minimally invasive bur anatomy. The bur tip is sharp and used for penetrating dense cortical bone. The body of the bur is often used in a seesaw motion to cut spongy cancellous bone. The smooth/inactive portion of the bur is highly important as this can be laid against skin or soft tissue without engagement which serves as protection when paired with irrigation.

The convergence/confluence of X ray, fluoroscopy, bur systems, along with technical innovations by surgeons, resulted in new standards of care across various subspecialties. The adoption of the bur system had a profound impact on modern foot surgery, expanding treatment options and revolutionizing the way procedures are performed today. Surgical burs allow for precise and controlled removal of bone and tissues as well as shaping of bones with higher finesse, while minimizing unnecessary damage to adjacent structures to reduce postoperative pain with improved cosmetic outcomes.

APPLICATIONS IN FOOT AND ANKLE SURGERY

MIS has significantly transformed foot and ankle surgery, providing many benefits over traditional open surgical techniques. Utilizing small incisions, specialized instruments, and advanced imaging technologies, MIS reduces tissue damage, minimizes scarring, and shortens recovery times. As aforementioned, this approach is advantageous as it decreases soft tissue trauma, periosteal stripping, and it allows the patient to recover faster. There are multiple applications for MIS in foot and ankle surgery. Traditional bunion surgery involves large incisions and substantial bone and soft tissue stripping and manipulation, leading to extended recovery periods and significant postoperative pain. In contrast, minimally invasive bunion surgery (MIBS) uses small incisions, less periosteal stripping, and realigns the big toe joint with minimal trauma. This offers not only a better cosmetic result; however, decreases the chance of scar tissue formation within the big toe joint which can lead to decreased postoperative range of motion.

Of note, there are now 6 iterations of MIBS. The first generation of MIBS began with the Reverdin-Isham procedure.[11] This technique was an adaptation of the traditional Reverdin osteotomy and involved MIS bone cuts using bur without internal or percutaneous fixation, relying on bandages for fixation. This technique is still practiced today; however, complications involve displacement/malunion (16%), shortening (4–6 mm), and stiffness.[10–15]

The second generation of MIBS saw the introduction of techniques such as the Bösch and SERI (Simple, Effective, Rapid, Inexpensive) methods. This technique seeked to alleviate the problems/complications encountered with the first generation by supplementing the osteotomies with a percutaneous K-wire fixation to maintain reduction. However, complications involve malunion (69%), recurrence (38%), pin tract infections (13%), and stiffness (14%).[12–17]

The third generation of MIBS, and the most impactful for creating a baseline of this method/construct, involves osseous first metatarsal bone cuts (chevron) using a bur, supplemented by stable internal fixation in the form of two long compression screws.

The fourth generation of MIBS involves only a slight modification by using a transverse osteotomy (rather than chevron), also with fixated with two screws.[18] The next transformative iteration/advancement (fifth generation) is hallmarked by use of a single metatarsal screw fixation construct using a compressive or non-compressive neutral pitch screw that is combined with a chevron osteotomy.[19-26]

The sixth generation is also a single metatarsal screw construct that uses dual-zone neutral pitch screw fixation, however involves the rotationally-controlled Transveron™ osteotomy.[24] Despite surgical and technological advances, complications with a new technique without a surgical playbook are more prevalent, and some are exclusive to this time of surgery.[19,22,27]

In addition to bunion surgery, MIS techniques have gained popularity in procedures such as trauma, Charcot reconstruction, and flatfoot reconstruction. MIS and the development of minimally invasive plate osteosynthesis (MIPO) have significantly transformed the treatment of trauma in general but more specifically calcaneal fractures. Traditionally, calcaneal fractures required extensive open surgery (lateral extensile approach), which often resulted in large incisions, substantial soft tissue damage, and lengthy recovery periods increasing chances of skin necrosis. However, the advent of MIS and MIPO techniques has revolutionized this approach by utilizing small incisions (sinus tarsi approach) and specialized instruments/plates/screw guides to achieve precise fracture reduction with percutaneous fixation. As a result, patients experience less postoperative pain, shorter hospital stays, and faster recovery times, enabling a quicker return to normal activities.

Charcot reconstruction involves a mixture of adjacent joint arthrodesis, intraosseous fixation/beaming, anatomic realignment while preserving foot length. The advancements in minimally invasive surgical techniques and technology allow surgeons to perform selective joint preparation/fusion while reducing the surgical biological impact and without undergoing severe segmental bone loss/removal. The benefits continue as this reduced soft tissue disruption and preservation of periosteal blood supply leads to lower incidence of wound-related complications in an already immunocompromised patient population.

MINIMALLY INVASIVE IMPLANT TECHNOLOGY

The most notable changes occurred in forefoot surgery in regards to the treatment of hallux valgus which laid the foundation for the current paradigm shift away from open procedures. In 1981, Dr. Basil Helal enumerated over 150 open procedures to treat bunions.[27,28] During the same decade (80s / 90s), pioneers/early adopters in the field of MIS sought to apply the same principles to foot surgery.

Progress in the field of MIBS technique/generations required innovation in instrumentation and screw design given unconventional fixation spanning the first metatarsal obliquely, traversing the lateral cortex of the proximal metatarsal shaft to capture the laterally translated metatarsal head. A minimally invasive screw is one with a fully threaded shaft and a beveled head and a variety of designs have been commercialized (**Fig 5**).[19] The first design is compressive in nature, between the head and shaft. Another design involved a non-compressive neutral pitch between the head and shaft. A novel design developed by Dr. Neal Blitz is a dual-zone shaft screw (neutral non-compressive throughout) has pitched segments to match the anatomy of the bone being engaged.

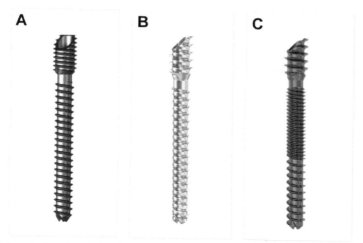

Fig. 5. Pitch variations in minimally invasive bunion screws that feature a beveled head and full threaded shaft. (*A*) Compressive pitch, (With permission from MI SCREW, Orthocape.) (*B*) Neutral, no-compression pitch, (*From* Revcon™ Neutra, Voom Medical Devices, Inc.) (*C*) Dual-zone neutral pitch, (*From* Revcon™ Anchor, Voom Medical Devices, Inc.).

Specific areas anatomic areas of interest where screw fixation engages the bone are as follows: The insertion point at the spongy proximal medial metatarsal shaft is coined the cancellous anchor zone (CAZ).[22] The lateral cortical wall of the first metatarsal is coined the cortical purchase zone (CPZ) and the distal insertion of the screw with the metatarsal head is coined the docking engagement zone (DEZ).[23] Each of these three contacts points contributes to the stability of the overall construct.

SUMMARY

In conclusion, the journey through the history of MIS in foot and ankle procedures reveals a remarkable narrative of innovation and progress. From the foundational discoveries of X rays and fluoroscopy, which paved the way for enhanced visualization and real-time imaging, to the evolution of surgical burs and the development of advanced techniques in foot surgery, each milestone has played a crucial role in reshaping the landscape of surgical practice. The adoption of atraumatic principles by surgeons further emphasizes the commitment to minimizing tissue damage and optimizing patient outcomes. The transformative impact of MIBS, spanning 3 generations of techniques, showcases a relentless pursuit of precision and efficiency. The incorporation of beveled screws in the latest generation stands as a testament to the ongoing biomechanical and research-driven advancements that contribute to the ultimate stability and success of minimally invasive procedures. As we reflect on this historical journey, it becomes evident that the fusion of technological innovation, surgical expertise, and patient-centric approaches has propelled minimally invasive foot surgery into a new era of excellence, offering patients improved outcomes and faster recovery.

CLINICS CARE POINTS

- Low speed high torque bur systems are preferred for minimally invasive surgery to avoid skin and bone burns.

- Shannon burs are ideal for precise osteotomies and wedge burs are ideal for destructive resections and joint arthrodesis.
- Specialized beveled headed screws should be used for most minimally invasive procedures depending on the indication.

DISCLOSURE

Vice President, Surgeon Education, Training & Onboarding—Voom Medical Devices, which is a paid position.

REFERENCES

1. Schollmeyer T, Soyinka AS, Schollmeyer M, et al. Georg Kelling (1866-1945): the root of modern day minimal invasive surgery. A forgotten legend? Arch Gynecol Obstet 2007;276:505–9.
2. Hatzinger M, Kwon ST, Langbein S, et al. Hans Christian Jacobaeus: inventor of human laparoscopy and thoracoscopy. J Endourol 2006;20:848–50.
3. Moll FH, Marx FJ. A pioneer in laparoscopy and pelviscopy: Kurt Semm (1927–2003). J Endourol 2005;19(PMID 15865510):269.
4. Litynski GS. Kurt Semm and the Fight against skepticism: Endoscopic hemostasis, laparoscopic appendectomy, and semm's impact on the "laparoscopic revolution". JSLS 1986;2(3):309–13.
5. Bhattacharya K, Kurt S. A laparoscopic crusader. J Minimal Access Surg 2007;3:35–6.
6. Tubiana Wilhelm Conrad röntgen and the discovery of X-rays. Bull Acad Natl Med 1996;180(1):97–108.
7. Pamboukian S. "Looking radiant": science, photography and the X-ray craze of 1896. Victorian Rev 2001;56–74.
8. Hirshfeld JW Jr, Balter S, Brinker JA, et al. American College of Cardiology Foundation; American Heart Association/; HRS; SCAI; American College of Physicians Task Force on Clinical Competence and Training. ACCF/AHA/HRS/SCAI clinical competence statement on physician knowledge to optimize patient safety and image quality in fluoroscopically guided invasive cardiovascular procedures: a report of the American College of Cardiology Foundation/American Heart Association/American College of Physicians Task Force on Clinical Competence and Training. Circulation 2005 Feb 1;111(4):511–32. https://doi.org/10.1161/01.CIR.0000157946.29224.5D.
9. Mahant R, Agrawal SV, Kapoor S, et al. Milestones of dental history. CHRISMED J Health Res 2017;4(4):229–34.
10. Texhammar R, Colton C, Perren SM, et al. AO/ASIF Instruments and Implants : A Technical Manual. Completely rev. and enl. 2nd ed. Springer-Verlag; 1994. 9–32.
11. Isham SA. The Reverdin-Isham procedure for the correction of hallux abducto valgus. A distal metatarsal osteotomy procedure. Clin Podiatr Med Surg 1991;8(1):81–94.
12. Frigg A, Zaugg S, Maquieira G, et al. Stiffness and range of motion after minimally invasive chevron-akin and open scarf-akin procedures. Foot Ankle Int 2019;40(5):515–25.
13. Oliva F, Longo UG, Maffulli N. Minimally invasive hallux valgus correction. Orthop Clin North Am 2009;40(4):525–30.

14. Gadek A, Liszka H, Zalewski M. Comment on "midterm results and complications after minimally invasive distal metatarsal osteotomy for treatment of hallux valgus." Foot Ankle Int 2013;34(10):1464.
15. Biz C, Fosser M, Dalmau-Pastor M, et al. Functional and radiographic outcomes of hallux valgus correction by mini- invasive surgery with Reverdin-Isham and Akin percutaneous osteotomies: a longitudinal prospective study with a 48-month follow-up. J Orthop Surg Res 2016;11(1):157.
16. Bauer T, de Lavigne C, Biau D, et al. Percutaneous hallux valgus surgery: a prospective multicenter study of 189 cases. Orthop Clin North Am 2009;40(4):505–14.
17. Malagelada F, Sahirad C, Dalmau-Pastor M, et al. Minimally invasive surgery for hallux valgus: a systematic review of current surgical techniques. Int Orthop 2018. https://doi.org/10.1007/s00264-018-4138-x.
18. Lewis TL, Lau B, Alkhalfan Y, et al. Fourth-generation minimally invasive hallux valgus surgery with metaphyseal extra-articular transverse and Akin osteotomy (META): 12 Month clinical and radiologic results. Foot Ankle Int 2023;44(3):178–91.
19. Blitz NM. Game-changing new modern minimally invasive surgery. Foot Ankle Q 2020;31(4):181–91.
20. Blitz NM. New minimally invasive bunion surgery: easier said than done. Foot Ankle Surg: techn. Rep Cases 2023;3(4):2023–100288.
21. Blitz NM. Current concepts in minimally invasive bunion surgery. Podiatry Today 2019;32(2).
22. Blitz NM, Wong DT, Baskin ES. Patterns of metatarsal explosion after new modern minimally invasive bunion surgery. A retrospective review and case series of 16 feet. J Min Invasive Bunion Surg. 2024;1:92774. https://doi.org/10.62485/001c.92774.
23. Blitz NM, Grecea B, Wong DT, et al. Defining the cortical purchase zone in new minimally invasive bunion surgery. A retrospective study of 638 cases. J Min Invasive Bunion Surg. 2024;1:92777. https://doi.org/10.62485/001c.92777.
24. Voom Medical Devices, Co. Revcon minimally invasive screw system surgical technique. Available at: https://www.voommedicaldevices.com/files/2023_Voom_OpTech_Complete_Digital_01.pdf.
25. Wong DT. A new paradigm for failed bunions with minimally invasive methods. Clin Podiatr Med Surg 2025;42(1):102–16.
26. Blitz NM. New minimally invasive bunion surgery: the End-all Be-all bunion repair? Clin Podiatr Med Surg 2025;42(1):10–31.
27. Di Nucci KA. The unfamiliar complications of minimally invasive foot surgery. Clin Podiatr Med Surg 2025;42(1):117–38.
28. Helal B. Surgery for adolescent hallux valgus. Clin Orthop Relat Res 1981;157:50–63.

New Minimally Invasive Bunion Surgery
The End-All Be-All Bunion Repair?

Neal M. Blitz, DPM[a,b,]*

KEYWORDS

- Minimally invasive bunion surgery
- Fifth generation minimally invasive bunion surgery
- Sixth generation minimally invasive bunion surgery • Transveron™
- Single screw minimally invasive bunion surgery • MIBS

KEY POINTS

- Patients are seeking a minimally invasive bunion solution that allows improved cosmesis and a functional walking recovery.
- Minimally Invasive Bunion Surgery (MIBS) is an accepted method of bunion repair for bunions of all severities.
- The current MIBS iteration (fifth and sixth generation) calls for a 1-screw construct and stabilizing osteotomy configuration. A fifth generation MIBS involves a chevron osteotomy paired with a single compressive or non-compressive MI screw. A sixth generation MIBS involves a Transveron™ osteotomy paired with a single dual-zone neutral pitched MI screw.
- Research and early meta-analyses data suggest MIBS is comparable (and improved) to traditional bunion surgery on radiographic/clinical outcomes.

INTRODUCTION

Bunion surgery is in the midst of undergoing a seismic paradigm shift to a new gold standard, and that is to new minimally invasive bunion surgery (MIBS).[1–5] Just like other orthopedic specialties that are downsizing incisions for improved outcomes and patient recoveries, the same transformation is rapidly happening in the foot and ankle community, with hallux valgus correction leading the way. New MIBS adequately addresses the major crucial pain points for both patients and surgeons, making it the best solution for bunion repair today and perhaps the "end-all be-all" bunion repair method.

---

[a] Private Practice, Blitz Footcare, 800A 5th Avenue, Suite 403, New York, NY 10065, USA;
[b] Private Practice, Blitz Footcare, 435 N. Roxbury Drive, Penthouse, Beverly Hills, CA 90210, USA
* Private Practice, Blitz Footcare, 800A 5th Avenue, Suite 403, New York, NY 10065.
E-mail address: drblitz@drnealblitz.com

Clin Podiatr Med Surg 42 (2025) 11–31
https://doi.org/10.1016/j.cpm.2024.09.004   **podiatric.theclinics.com**

Bunion surgery as an overall procedure has a historical negative perception for both surgeons and patients due to the wide variety of corrective options, invasiveness, significant downtime/disability, complications, and often unappealing cosmetic result.[1] As such, both parties may delay surgical repair for as long as humanly possible or simply avoid the surgery altogether. New MIBS is revolutionary as it involves a fluoroscopic-assisted "laparoscopic-like approach" that allows for a structural osseous bone realignment repair performed through tiny incisions/portals and permits an immediate walking recovery.[2,4–6] Once surgeons become proficient in minimally invasive (MI) bunion correction, the results have seemingly improved outcomes/cosmesis and a functional walking recovery.[7–10] The benefits of MIBS are listed in **Box 1**.

This "new" technique is revolutionary as it relies on transformative bony realignment and regeneration, rather than correction-limiting bone cuts/wedges or force-fusing joint(s) of the foot. The procedure involves a brand-new osteotomy realignment and fixation construct, all performed with new instrumentation (low-speed high-torque rotary burs) and specialized MIBS-specific implant (screw) technology. The procedure calls for a distally based subcapital first metatarsal osteotomy whereby the metatarsal head (and sesamoids, as a unit) is disconnected from its proximal segment, then significantly shifted/realigned into a corrected position that is fixated with 1 or 2 MI screw(s) (**Figs. 1** and **2**). The resultant construct leaves little to no bone-to-bone contact between bony segments, whereby the fixation screws often span a large osseous void. Over the course of the 6 to 12 weeks recovery, the body naturally regenerates the first metatarsal bone to fill-in the osseous defect, eventually producing a straight metatarsal.[11] This version of MIBS can be used to treat bunions of all sizes/severities with a walking recovery in surgical shoe, also allowing for same day bilateral correction. Research and literature have emerged from MIBS innovators and early adopters that not only support these methods and new technology as an acceptable bunion correction but also as a new soon-to-be worldwide standard in bunion surgery.

THE DOWNSIDES OF EXISTING BUNION SURGERY METHODS

With nearly 2 centuries having passed since the first bunionectomy (exostectomy) was published (Dr Gernet 1836) and over 150 different procedures for surgeons to choose from, it is no wonder that there is still no consensus on the best method to treat this first metatarsal misalignment.[12] The available surgical "bunionectomy" options have involved soft tissue release(s), bumpectomy, realignment/wedge osteotomy, joint fusion, or a combination thereof.[13–15] Surgeons have relied on angular radiographic measurements as a guideline for procedure selection, which is mainly a function of bunion severity.[16,17] Frontal plane position has become a topic of debate and focus in the last decade.[18] Small bunions would be indicated for a distally based procedure (most likely a metatarsal osteotomy) in close proximity to the big toe joint. Large

---

Box 1
Benefits of new minimally invasive bunion surgery (MIBS)

Laparoscopic-like with tiny incisions (improved cosmesis)

Immediate weightbearing in postop shoe

Hardware internal to the bone

Preserves motion (avoids fusion)

Quells hypermobility

Allows for same day bilateral surgery

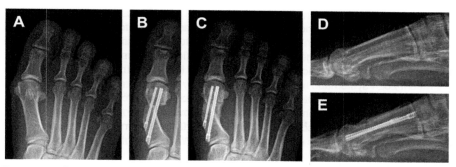

Fig. 1. MIBS for moderate bunion using "classically described" 2-screw construct. (*A, D*) Preoperative radiographs demonstrating bunion deformity with the displacement of the sesamoids. (*B*) Postoperative radiograph at 2 weeks after MIBS with 2-screw construct. The screws span an osseous defect that was created as a result of the translation/realignment. (*C, E*) Postoperative radiographs at 3 months reveal exuberant callus formation with a resultant regenerated straight first metatarsal bone. On the lateral, the subcapital osteotomy line/lucency can still be identified and will fully consolidate/fade over several months. (Image courtesy of David T. Wong, DPM.)

bunions, on the other hand, seemed to have been best suited for a proximally based solution with either a metatarsal osteotomy close to the tarsometatarsal joint or a midfoot fusion. However, surgeon-specific experience trumps these so-called guidelines whereby surgeons generally rely on their own playbook for procedure selection, even if it contradicts angular guideline norms.[19]

Despite the smorgasbord of surgical solutions, the overall complication rate and recurrence rate remain staggeringly high for traditional bunion surgery, making operative repair somewhat of an unpredictable or unreliable solution.[20–22] A systematic review of 229 hallux valgus studies published in the *Journal of Bone and Joint Surgery* by Barg and

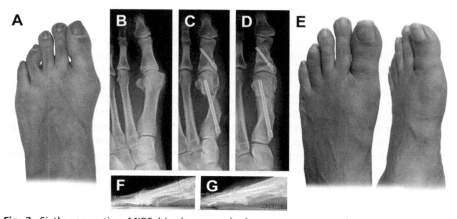

Fig. 2. Sixth generation MIBS (single screw dual-zone construct and Transveron™ osteotomy) for a mild bunion. (*A, B, F*) Preoperative clinical and radiographs demonstrating bunion deformity. (*C*) Postoperative radiograph at 2 weeks after subcapital first metatarsal osteotomy fixated with a single screw (dual-zone) and an adjunctive Akin osteotomy. The screw spans an osseous defect that was created as a result of the translation/realignment. (*D, E, G*) Postoperative radiographs at 3.5 months reveal exuberant callus formation with a resultant regenerated straight first metatarsal bone and realigned sesamoids/hallux. The tiny incisional portals are nearly invisible.

colleagues identified a patient dissatisfaction rate of 10.6%, postoperative big toe joint pain of 1.5%, and a recurrence of 4.9%.[23] A meta-analysis performed by Ezzatvar and colleagues (2021) of 2914 individuals among 23 studies identified a 25% recurrence rate after open bunion surgery.[24] There is a significant inconsistency in terminology and categorization of complications associated with hallux valgus surgery as evidenced in a recent 2024 systematic review of 142 studies by AlMeshari and colleagues. Recurrence was mentioned in 54% of studies and nonunion in 53%.[25] The complication rate after various Lapidus fixation procedures was as low as 13% (plantar-plating) and as high as 24.5% (screws), according to a current (2024) systematic review and meta-analysis involving 16 studies (1176 participants).[26] While each of the traditional surgical techniques has its benefits for certain bunion criteria, there has yet to be a method that has universal applicability across the ranges of bunion severities.

Modified McBride

Soft tissue procedures and bumpectomy (McBride procedure) as an isolated bunion solution are generally avoided, particularly as bunion severity increases.[27] Small bunions with minimal angular deformity, with more of a medial eminence projection, can be indicated for exostectomy with or without lateral release. The recurrence rate of isolated McBride Bunionectomy has been reported as 72.2%.[28] One benefit of exostectomy is the simplicity of the procedure, limited downtime, and walking recovery. This approach is beneficial as it generally does not "burn any bridges" for a future osteotomy procedure so long as the exostectomy was not too invasive/destructive to the big toe joint.

Open Distal Metatarsal Osteotomy

Incisional (or open) distal metatarsal osteotomy is currently the most common approach for mild to moderate bunions, in the absence of pathologic hypermobility.[29,30] An Austin/chevron-based intracapsular osteotomy of the first metatarsal head through a dorsal medial or medial incision fixated by 1 or 2 screws has been the most reproducible approach.[31–34] The extent of correction is dictated by the amount of bone overlap of the cancellous portion of the osteotomy while obtaining a rigid internal structural fixation. Some osteotomy variations (long arm Austin) have allowed for greater bone shifts and, therefore, incrementally larger bunion correction.[35] Specific complications to distal metatarsal osteotomies are recurrence, malunion, shortening, hallux varus, and/or arthrofibrosis.[36,37]

Open Midshaft Osteotomy

These diaphyseal-heavy osteotomies are effective at addressing moderate and large bunions while also permitting a walking recovery due to the inherent structural configuration of the cut and hardware placement. They are more complex to perform, have a large incisional component, and have been criticized for comparatively slower healing of the cortical diaphyseal bone portion(s) of the osteotomy.[38] The most notable of the midshaft osteotomy is the Scarf osteotomy, which is criticized for correctional loss due to troughing. The advantages of Scarf over distal osteotomy remain a subject of investigation.[39] The Scarf continues to be prevalent in Europe (being replaced by MIBS), but in the United States midshaft osteotomies were replaced by Lapidus-fusion procedures.

Incisional Proximal Metatarsal Osteotomy/Wedges

Incisional osteotomies and wedges of the metatarsal base have fallen out of favor as they have also been replaced by Lapidus-type midfoot fusion procedures.[40,41] While metatarsal base corrections are excellent at angular realignment through various bone cuts and wedges, they are structurally unstable with weightbearing (despite fixation methods) and, therefore, require a miserable protracted patient recovery experience involving large boots, casts, and/or crutches.

Lapidus-type Fusion

Open incisional first tarsometatarsal joint arthrodesis and its variations have been the seemingly preferred bunion repair method for larger angular deformities in the past 2 decades, particularly in the United States.[42–46] Surgeons who believe bunions occur as a result of tarsometatarsal joint failure (hypermobility) advocate repositioning the entire first metatarsal bone through the midfoot fusion joint complex that corrects both the angular misalignment and bunion-causing instability.[47] Advances in tarsometatarsal-specific orthopedic hardware and surgical techniques have dramatically lessened the fusion-nonunion rate to less than 10%, which has comparatively been considered an acceptable complication rate.[43,48–50] Additionally, early weightbearing protocols have lessened the crutch-time dependency and removable knee-high boots have replaced casts, which has made the surgery much more palatable to patients.[43,44,46] Incisions have become "smaller" with guided instrumentation Lapidus jigs and/or spanning-joint fusion nails, both providing some cosmetic benefit to patients through smaller incisions. With all these technological advances, Lapidus surgery still permanently removes one's natural joint anatomy/function and carries a significant postoperative recovery/downtime (6–8 weeks of large boots/casts and/or crutches), thereby limiting the widespread use of this procedure for all bunions.

Big Toe Joint Fusion

Eliminating the big toe joint for bunion treatment should have extreme narrow indications of significant painful arthritis, unreducible/ankylosed hallux valgus, large/severe deformity, advanced age, and/or necessitating medical comorbidities.[48–51] While the surgery is effective at realigning the big toe, it eliminates the propulsive nature of the foot, and therefore, in the authors opinion should be a last resort. Moreover, combining Lapidus-type fusion and first metatarsophalangeal joint fusion doubly removes the first ray mobility and a patient's propulsive gait.[52] It is the authors opinion that these "double fusions" should also be avoided unless a last resort.[53] Joint fusion of the locomotive ball and socket complex of the big toe joint is not an ideal solution for the bunion patient.

MINIMALLY INVASIVE BUNION SURGERY EVOLUTION

Minimally incision surgery has evolved since its introduction, and it is important to understand that not all MIBS is the same.[54] For the context of bunion surgery and specifically, the acronym "MIBS" refers to a fluoroscopically assisted realignment subcapital first osteotomy (using low-speed high-torque rotary burs) fixated by long scaffolding fully threaded beveled headed screw(s) all performed through small, tiny laparoscopic-like incisions (<1.5 cm). What is not considered MIBS is any open method where large incisions become smaller and formal dissection occurs, as true minimally invasive surgery is considered dissection-free. Moreover, "minimally invasive" intramedullary plating or percutaneous Lapidus-fusions should also not be confused or mislabeled as MIBS.

Minimally invasive bunion surgery morphed from simple unfixated percutaneous bumpectomies to advanced osteotomies and innovative screw fixation allowing for major first ray deformity correction. The evolution of each iteration has been collectively referred to as "generations."[1] The first generation involved intracapsular osteotomy of the first metatarsal head with bandage splinting (Isham, 1991).[55] The second generation involved a transverse first metatarsal neck osteotomy with a percutaneous positional axial stabilizing K-wire (Bösch 1990, Giannini 2008).[56,57] The third generation, and most transformative advancement, involves a subcapital chevron osteotomy fixated by two parallel percutaneous chamfered headed fully threaded screw fixation (Redfern & Vernois, 2013).[2] The fourth generation slightly differs from its predecessor generation by substituting a transverse flat-cut osteotomy (rather than a chevron) (Lewis et al, 2023).[58,59] The next transformative iteration/advancement (fifth and sixth generation) is hallmarked by use of a single metatarsal screw (1-screw) fixation construct that is combined with a stabilizing osteotomy configuration (Blitz 2023).[1,4,9,60,61] The differentiation between the fifth and sixth generations are based on the osteotomy type and type of MIBS screw used. The fifth generation involves either a single compressive or non-compressive neutral pitched screw fixation with a chevron osteotomy, whereas the sixth generation involves a single dual-zone neutral pitch screw fixation with a Transveron™ osteotomy.

FIRST METATARSAL REGENERATION

The newness of MIBS and the unfamiliar shift/realignment and fixation construct leaving a large bony defect has many surgeons questioning if and how the bone will heal. A novel retrospective study by the author (Blitz and colleagues) in 172 feet after MIBS classified and characterized the lateral bone healing (first metatarsal regeneration— FMR).[11] We specifically evaluated the triangular region of the lateral metatarsal where bone healing occurs (termed the regeneration triangle) (**Fig. 3**). Three types of FMR healing were identified, using the primary screw as a demaraction line to discern medial from lateral healing (**Fig. 4**). Type I FMR occurred only medial to the primary screw (17.4%). Type II FMR occurred both medial and just lateral to the primary screw (42.4%), and Type III FMR occurred robustly (exuberant) all around the primary screw (40.1%). All the 3 FMR types are acceptable healing, and it should be noted that 82.5% of feet had healing also lateral to the primary screw. Importantly this study included bunions of all sizes with a mean preoperative intermetatarsal angle IMA of 15.8° (smallest IMA was 12.1° and largest was 19.5°), though there was no significant correlation to a FMR type. A majority of cases (85%) involved 1-screw MIBS and given this heavily weighted cohort, no statistical correlation between the number of screws and the FMR type was achieved.

FIFTH AND SIXTH GENERATION MINIMALLY INVASIVE BUNION SURGERY

The benefits of a 1-screw construct are significant to the patient, surgeon, and to the health care system with a lower cost to deliver care (**Box 2**). Below outlines several factors and several aspects/components that should be taken into account when considering a single metatarsal screw, as the screw alone is not the only factor creating a stable 1-screw MIBS construct.

Stabilizing Osteotomy Configurations

Being that MIBS allows for a surgeon-dictated walking recovery, there is an increased risk for capital fragment positional loss when weightbearing without a second point of fixation. A 1-screw fixation construct, by itself, is susceptible to unwanted metatarsal head rotation/displacement, and this risk can be mitigated with a stabilizing osteotomy that acts as an additional point of fixation. The transverse osteotomy, by design, is not suitable for a 1-screw construct (with weightbearing) as there is no interlocking nature to this flat-smooth cut. Below describes 2 stabilizing osteotomies that would create a secondary point of osseous fixation to counteract rotational instability.

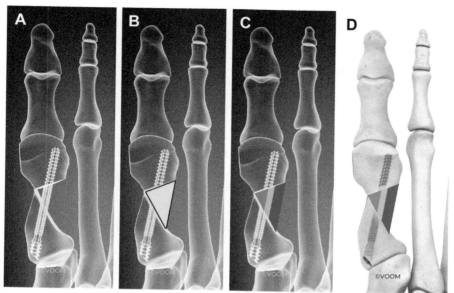

Fig. 3. Rendering illustrating the regeneration triangle and types of FMR. (*A*) MIBS demonstrating 1-screw construct. (*B*) The regeneration triangle (*yellow*) is the available area for bone healing. (*C, D*) Types of FMR healing using the primary (anchor) screw as a reference to assess medial and lateral callus formation. Type I FMR (*red*), Type II (*blue*), and Type III (*purple*). (*From* Blitz NM, Wong DT, Grecea B, Baskin ES. Characterization of First Metatarsal Regeneration After New Modern Minimally Invasive Bunion Surgery. A Retrospective Radiographic Review of 172 Cases. J Min Invasive Bunion Surg. 2024;1. doi:10.62485/001c.92756.)

Chevron

This is the most iconic metatarsal osteotomy in the history of bunion surgery and also the basis of the third generation MIBS. The "V" configuration is an inherently very stable interlocking design that only permits one plane of motion along the axis of the apex, and in the case of bunion surgery that is in the transverse plane to achieve inter-metatarsal angular correction. Because of this restrictive nature of the configuration, the chevron cut does not allow for any rotatory sesamoid correction but also protects from unwanted rotation as well. The chevron is a constrained or rotationally-blocked osteotomy, and is suitable for a 1-screw construct. A fifth generation MIBS involves a chevron osteotomy paired with a single compressive or non-compressive MI screw.

Transveron™[a,b]

A new osteotomy designed and configured specifically for MIBS. As the name "Transveron™" describes, it is a combination of the benefits of the chevron and transverse configurations without the negatives of each configuration. The transverse portion of the osteotomy is dorsal and lateral, and the chevron plantar-medial. This allows for both metatarsal head lateral translation and rotational freedom with a small shelf of stability to resist the dorsal displacement risk associated with weightbearing. The Transveron™ is ideal for a 1-screw MIBS construct

---

[a] Provisional Patent Application: No. 63/454,005 filed on 3-22-2023

[b] Non Provisional Patent: US App 18/518,376 filed 3-22-2024

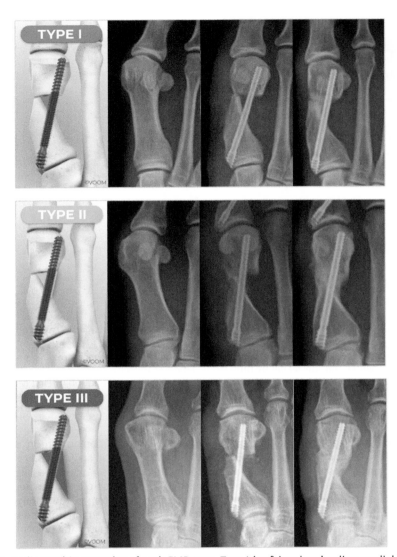

Fig. 4. Radiographic examples of each FMR type. Type I (*red*) involves healing medial to the primary screw. Type II (*blue*) represents both medial and lateral healing around the screw fixation. Type III (*purple*) is characterized by exuberant robust bone formation throughout. (*Modified from* Blitz NM, Wong DT, Grecea B, Baskin ES. Characterization of First Metatarsal Regeneration After New Modern Minimally Invasive Bunion Surgery. A Retrospective Radiographic Review of 172 Cases. J Min Invasive Bunion Surg. 2024;1:92756. https://doi.org/10.62485/001c.92756.)

as it is rotationally-controlled and not constrained (compared with the chevron). A sixth generation MIBS involves a Transveron™ osteotomy paired with a single dual-zone neutral pitched MI screw.

Anchor Screw Stability and Placement

All MIBS requires fixational stability to maintain osseous realignment correction while bony regeneration occurs.[11] The most important stability providing MIBS fixation

Box 2
Benefits of single screw minimally invasive bunion surgery (MIBS) (fifth generation MIBS)
Less internal hardware
Technically easier perform
Quicker operative time
Less incisions/cosmesis
Increased medial ledge resection
Lower risk of bur-induced nerve injury
Possible less metatarsal explosion risk
Overall health care delivery cost savings

component is the primary screw (a.k.a., anchor screw).[9] The second screw in the constructs (a.k.a., collateral screw) main purpose is to counteract rotational stability, though this function can also be achieved with a stabilizing osteotomy configuration (chevron or Transveron™). The chevron is rotationally-locked whereas the Transveron™ is rotationally-controlled. Nonetheless, MIBS can be achieved with a 1-screw construct, however, the stability/strength of the construct is partially dictated by the placement of the anchor screw.

There are 3 anatomic locations for MIBS anchor screw stability, which are located within[1]: the medial first metatarsal base (Cancellous Anchor Zone—CAZ),[2] the lateral cortical wall of the first metatarsal (Cortical Purchase Zone—CPZ),[3] and the metatarsal head (Docking Engagement Zone—DEZ).[62] The location within the CPZ that the anchor screw exits/pierces the lateral cortex is considered a primary source of the constructs stability[9,62] (**Fig. 5**). The further distance the screw exits the CPZ from the osteotomy (termed the cortical runway) the more cortical real estate there is around the screw, which may be protective from developing fractures contiguous with the osteotomy and/or metatarsal explosion.[62] In a previous research study, performed by the author and colleagues, we defined and classified CPZ stability regions based on the statistical empirical rule involving 638 feet over a period of 5 years, starting with a single surgeon (N.M.B.) first and consecutive cases thereafter.[9] The mean anchor screw runway distance was 10.4±3.7 mm (95% CI, 10.1–10.7). A cortical runway distance less than 6.6 mm was considered to be more risky for fixation instability and considered a "no-go" zone as an anatomic location to preferably avoid. Conversely, a cortical runway distance greater than 14.2 mm would be considered more protective. It is inferred from this study that the lengthier the anchor screw cortical runway then the more stable the MIBS construct would be.

Novel Dual-Zone Minimally Invasive Bunion Surgery Screw

Minimally invasive bunion surgery requires a novel construct configuration where existing traditional orthopedic hardware could not meet the anatomical needs for fixating bony segments across a large void. This need gave rise to the chamfered head screw with a fully threaded shaft design (**Fig. 6**). The purpose of the MIBS screw(s) is to provide structural support and act as a metallic scaffold for bony ingrowth. The first MIBS screw that was developed has a compressive pitch between the head and the shaft. Alternative, neutral (no-compression) screws emerged to purely stabilize (rather than compress) the bony segments, acting only as a structural metallic scaffold for secondary bone healing callus. More recently, a dual-zone neutral pitch MIBS screw that has a shaft with a pitch that matches the bony densities for which that portion of the screw is engaging. The proximal aspect of the shaft has a

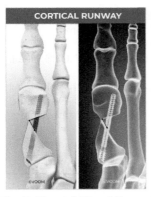
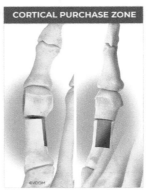
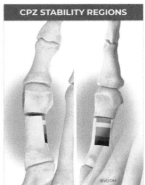

Fig. 5. The stability of the anchor screw is partially derived from where the screw engages the lateral first metatarsal cortex. The available area for the screw to capture the cortical wall is called the "Cortical Purchase Zone—CPZ (*pink*)." When the screw is in close proximity to the osteotomy then fixation destabilization and/or fracture can occur. The distance between the osteotomy and the screws exit within the CPZ is called the "Cortical Runway." The lengthier the distance/runway then the more cortical rim there is around the screw, which theorectically has a stabilizing effect. The CPZ stability region classification system (boundaries defined by the statistical empirical rule) might delineate stability based on distance from the osteotomy. The CPZ stability region boundaries have been defined as: danger (red, <2.9 mm), vulnerable (yellow, 3.0–6.6 mm), standard (green, 6.6–14.1 mm), safety (purple, 14.2–17.8 mm), and the security (blue, >17.9 mm). (*Modified from* Blitz NM, Grecea B, Wong DT, Baskin ES. Defining the Cortical Purchase Zone in New Minimally Invasive Bunion Surgery. A Retrospective Study of 638 Cases. J Min Invasive Bunion Surg. 2024;1:92777. https://doi.org/10.62485/001c.92777.)

tighter pitch to match the bone density of the CPZ. The distal end of the screw reverts back to a wider pitch to match the cancellous bone within the metatarsal head (DEZ). Structurally, this dual-zone configuration screw lends itself to 1-screw construct and is a construct-specific design for MIBS. A sixth generation MIBS involves a Transveron™ osteotomy paired with a single dual-zone neutral pitched MI screw.[60]

Medial Ledge Resection

A major advantage of a 1-screw MIBS construct is that it allows for greater medial ledge resection. The prominent bone on the medial aspect of the foot as a result of the MIBS translation is called the medial ledge, and the available bone for resection forms a triangular area (a term we coined, the medial ledge resection triangle [MLRT]) (**Fig. 7**). Any prominent redundant medial bone may become painful for patients, a sequalae/condition that we also coined as the "pseudobunion."[63] The presence of a second screw increases the propensity for a pseudobunion as more bony real estate is needed to insert that screw.

POSTOPERATIVE PROTOCOL

The industry standard with MIBS seems to be a weightbearing protocol in a postoperative shoe for 6 weeks. Of course, doctor-patient-specific protocols are determined by patient compliance, patient general and bone health, MIBS construct stability (osteotomy configuration, screw type, screw placement, and number of screws), and the extent of metatarsal head translation. At the 6-week mark, patients are generally transferred to stable shoe gear and an increase in activity is permitted. Bony

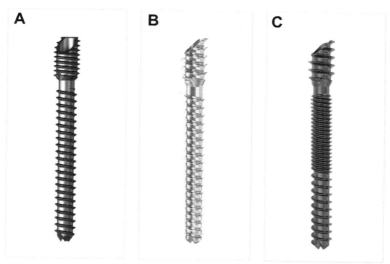

Fig. 6. Minimally invasive bunion surgery screws are fully threaded with a beveled head. (*A*) Compressive pitch between the head and shaft (*B*) Neutral (no-compression) between the head and shaft. Here the head of the screw has pitch modifications to the head to match the insertional cancellous bone of the first metatarsal base insertion point (*C*) Dual-zone screw with neutral pitch throughout that matches the density of the intended bone that is engaged. The tighter cortical pitch of the shaft is meant to engage the denser cortical bone of the lateral wall. The wider cancellous pitch of the end (tip) is meant to engage the spongy bone of the metatarsal head. A (With permission from MI SCREW, Orthocape.) B (From: Revcon™ Neutra, Voom Medical Devices, Inc.) C (From: Revcon™ Anchor, Voom Medical Devices, Inc.)

regenerate may be seen at this stage within the regenerative triangle; however, the decision to transition shoe gear and/or activities is often based on the clinical scenario (pain/discomfort and/or swelling), provided the radiographs are not suspicious for something that might preclude transition. Typically, at 3 months patients have returned to full activity without limitations. Swelling has decreased dramatically by this period postop, though full edema resolution may take 6 months to a year.

MINIMALLY INVASIVE BUNION SURGERY SPECIFIC COMPLICATIONS

No surgery is immune to postoperative complications, and MIBS has its fair share sequelae.[63] However, in comparison to many of the complications of traditional bunion surgery, MIBS complications are significantly lessened in frequency. Due to the laparoscopic portal-like incisions with MIBS, infection rates (cellulitis/osteomyelitis) are decreased without the large open/exposed nature of open bunionectomy. Bunion recurrence rates are low and under 1%.[5] Hallux varus incidence is also lower a possible occurence after any bunion surgery method. Minimally Invasive specific complications have come to the forefront as well as brand-new never been seen before complications. Symptomatic plantarflexory malunion of the capital fragment occurs mostly as a MIBS inexperienced issue. Similarly, incisional bur-burn wounds becomes nearly inexistent with experience and knowing when to excise skin-damaged portals. Consistent and constant irrigation while the bur is in use will additionally limit/prevent thermal injuries to the skin, soft tissue, and bone. Heat necrosis may be contributing factors to nonunion and/or osteomyelitis. Though radiographic

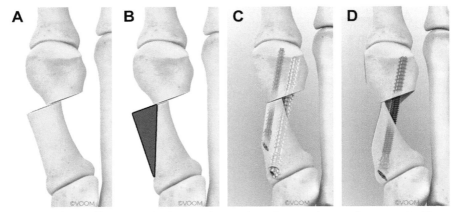

Fig. 7. Rendering illustrating the impact the number of screws has on the amount of bone that could be resected. (*A*) After lateral translation of the metatarsal head and medial toppling of the proximal metatarsal. (*B*). The available bone for resection is represented at a triangular area on the medial redundant metatarsal shaft, called the "Medial Ledge Resection Triangle—MLRT (brown triangle)." (*C*) A 2-screw MIBS construct shrinks the MLRT, reducing the amount of bone that could be resected due to the interference of the collateral screw. (*D*) A 1-screw MIBS construct allows for greater removal (if not the entire) prominent medial ledge, thereby reducing the risk of pseudobunion. (*From* Voom Medical Devices, Inc; With permission.)

nonunion is not uncommon and should not be treated unless unstable with persistent symptoms (pain and swelling) that have failed noninvasive methods to stimulate ossification/regeneration (ie, bone stimulator).

Bur-related nerve issues are possible whenever nerve structures are in close proximity to the bur. Removing the medial ledge places the dorsal medial cutaneous nerve at-risk with many proximally based resection techniques. Pseudobunion (a term coined by the author) is a new, never been described before sequela and lessened with a 1-screw method and adequate resection of the medial ledge. Also, a new recently described uncommon MIBS complication is metatarsal explosion (various fractures involving the CPZ) with and without displacement and/or loss of correction.[62] While radiographically violent appearing, metatarsal explosion is often managed without reoperation and heal inconsequentially. Though MIBS experience and best practices/advanced techniques are thought to lessen the risk, the authors have stated metatarsal explosion is "inevitable."[62]

MINIMALLY INVASIVE BUNION SURGERY OUTCOMES

In the context of bunion surgery, MIBS remains a relatively "new" bunion procedure and for a long time may have been considered "quackery" and/or an unaccepted method of repair. Just recently in September 2024, the American Orthopedic Society of Foot & Ankle Surgeons (AOFAS) released a positional statement by the Evidence Based Medicine Committee whereby AOFAS "endorses minimally invasive surgery [MIBS] as an option for the correction of mild to moderately severe hallux valgus deformity. We do not consider this procedure to be experimental."[64] The basis for the position change has been the many research studies demonstrating safety and effectiveness of MIBS at repairing hallux valgus deformity. The utility of MIBS for bunions of all sizes can be seen in **Figs. 8–13**.

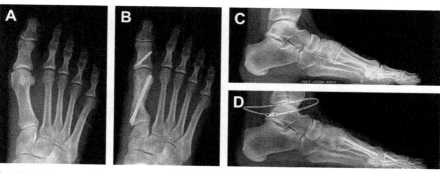

Fig. 8. Sixth generation MIBS (single screw dual-zone construct and Transveron™ osteotomy) for mild bunion. (*A, C*) Preoperative radiographs reveal the deformity. (*B, D*) Postoperative radiographs at 3 months after MIBS and adjunctive Akin procedure. A single dual-zone screw was used in the metatarsal. Robust FMR Type III bone healing is evident with a resultant straight metatarsal and corrected bunion. On the lateral view (*D*), the screw is ideally placed centrally within the metatarsal canal.

A landmark *Journal of Bone & Joint* (2021, Lewis and colleagues) single-surgeon third generation MIBS cases series of 292 feet with a 2-year follow-up demonstrated statistically significant improvements in patient satisfaction scores, visual analog pain scores, and radiographic parameters.[5] The mean intermetatarsal angle decreased from 18.2° to 6.3°, also demonstrating the utility for large bunion deformities. A separate study by Lewis and colleagues involving 59 third generation MIBS and 3-year follow-up demonstrated a 76.8% patient satisfaction rate along with statistically significant radiographic angular correction.[65] Neufeld and colleagues assessed a surgeon's first 94 third generation MIBS procedures with 94% of patients reporting good or excellent satisfaction with the procedure, despite the learning curve of the procedure.[66] Holme and colleagues performed a consecutive series of 40 patients undergoing third generation MIBS with 70% of patients reporting excellent outcomes and 30% reporting good

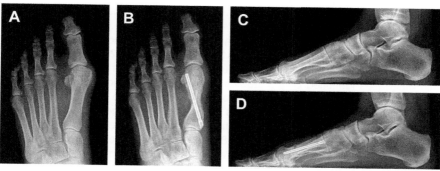

Fig. 9. Sixth generation MIBS (single screw dual-zone construct and Transveron™ osteotomy) for moderate bunion with a long metatarsal. (*A, C*) Preoperative radiographs exhibit the hallux valgus deformity with a long first metatarsal, enlarged medial eminence, and lateral adaption of the first metatarsophalangeal joint articular surface. (*B, D*) Postoperative radiographs at 3 months after MIBS fixated 1-screw construct with a dual-zone screw. The cartilage of the first metatarsal head is now rectus, which was corrected by slightly abducting the capital fragment prior to fixation. Also, resection of the prominent medial metatarsal head bunion region allows the hallux to site rectus on the metatarsal head. The regenerative triangle demonstrates FMR Type II.

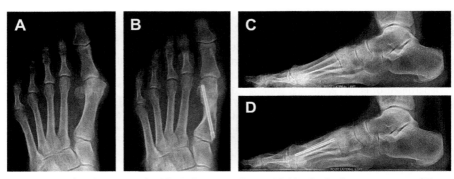

Fig. 10. Large bunion treated with sixth generation MIBS (single dual-zone screw and Trans-veron™ osteotomy). (*A, C*) Preoperative radiographs demonstrate the subluxation of the sesamoids within the interspace. (*B, D*) Postoperative radiographs at 6 months show a fully regenerated and straight first metatarsal bone. The frontal plane was corrected by rotating the capital fragment to realign the sesamoids. The sesamoids are nicely realigned below the first metatarsal head and the prominent medial eminence was resected flush. The lateral demonstrates a perfectly aligned first metatarsal head with the proximal metatarsal shaft.

outcomes, with various standard reporting questionnaires/scores.[67] No recurrence was identified at 12 months, and there were no major complications.

Narcotic usage after MIBS is significantly decreased as a result of the MI nature of the procedure and important consideration in the setting of an opioid epidemic. A national database query study by Granadillo identified about 21% hallux valgus corrective surgery had prolonged postoperative narcotic usage.[68] A comparative single center prospective study (Caolo and colleagues) evaluating narcotic usage after MI bunion correction versus incisional Lapidus or Scarf.[69] The narcotic usage was statistically significant with the Lapidus/Scarf cohort consuming 11 times the amount of pills. MIBS patients average 2.5 opioid pills and no medication refill requests. Mikhail and colleagues retrospectively demonstrated a patient satisfaction rate of 91.6% in 274 feet.[70] Their study also tracked narcotic usage and the mean postoperative oxycodone consumption was 2.2 pills.

Due to the evolution of MIBS and varying techniques and fixation constructs comparative analysis between studies has been challenging. In 2009, Roukis T.S. performed a systematic review of percutaneous osteotomies within a wide range of electronic databases identified only 3 studies of acceptable methodological quality (all involving unfixated osteotomies).[71] Due to the limited data, no recommendation for or against percutaneous osteotomies was made. In 2019, Malgelada and colleagues similarly attempted to perform a systematic review on MI surgery (first, second, and third generation techniques), reviewed 278 articles with 23 meeting inclusion criteria (2279 procedures in 1762 patients). There were "too few studies on each surgical technique category to assess whether one [MIBS generation] is more effective that the rest" and "too little evidence to allow for data pooling or meta-analysis."[72]

With the increasing use of internal fixation for MI bunion treatment, more high-quality research studies emerged making comparative studies more reliable. A 2020 meta-analysis publication of 11 studies with 1166 MI cases and 1035 open traditional bunionectomy cases revealed a significantly higher radiographic angular improvement with the MI group. Patient-reported outcomes were similar although the authors warned that pooled data threatened the validity of their observations.[11] In 2022, a MI versus open surgery hallux valgus meta-analysis was performed

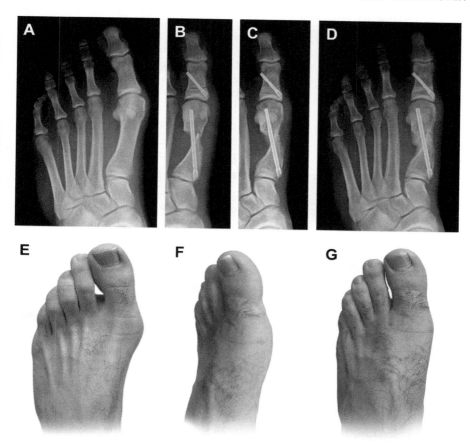

Fig. 11. Clinical and radiographic healing series after sixth generation MIBS. (*A*) Preoperative radiograph with hallux valgus and hallux interphalangeus. There is resultant lateral flattening (adaption) of the articular surface from the longstanding bunion. (*B*) Postoperative radiograph at 3 weeks after MIBS with a single dual-zone screw in the metatarsal and an adjunctive Akin. A Transveron™ osteotomy was performed and is an additional point of fixation at the metatarsal head/metatarsal shaft interface. Also, note the reduction/realignment of the sesamoids with frontal plane rotation and corrective angulation of the head to reorient the articular cartilage. Using a sixth generation MIBS (single dual-zone construct and stabilizing rotationally-controlled Transveron™ osteotomy allows for almost complete removal of the medial ledge. (*C*) Postoperative radiograph at 6 weeks reveals callus forming within the first metatarsal regeneration triangle. (*D*) Postoperative radiograph at 3 months with FMR Type III and a rectus first metatarsophalangeal joint. Removing the significant medial ledge eliminates the "bent" appearance of the healed metatarsal as well as reduces the risk for pseudobunion. (*E*) Preoperative clinical (top view) demonstrates the bunion and hallux abutting the second toe.(*F*) Postoperative healed clinical (side view) and (*G*) postoperative healed clinical (top view) are impressive as the incisional portals cannot even be identified.

involving 22 studies with 790 MI-treated feet and 838 openly treated feet. While this study included several generations of MIBS, as whole the authors concluded that the "MI procedures were more effective than open surgeries in the treatment of hallux valgus" and the "MI group achieved better radiologic and clinical outcomes compared with the open group."[73] A systematic review for recurrent bunions treated

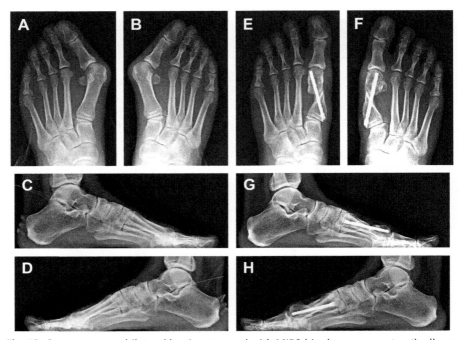

Fig. 12. Severe extreme bilateral bunions treated with MIBS (single screw construct), all performed on the same operative date. (*A, D*) Preoperative radiographs of the left foot and (*B, C*) preoperative radiographs of the right foot, both reveal severe bunions with very long first metatarsal bone. The sesamoids are very much rotated into the interspace on both feet, along with lateral cartilage adaption of the first metatarsal head. Postoperative radiographs of the left foot (*E, H*) and postoperative radiographs of the right foot (*F, G*) reveal a dramatic MIBS transformation. First metatarsal length was corrected by shortening angulation of the osteotomy to restore the parabola on both feet. The entire medial ledge was entirely resected, made possible by a 1-screw construct and stabilizing osteotomy. The sesamoids were realigned beneath the metatarsal head, and the cartilage was rectus allowing for a congruent first metatarsophalangeal joint. Type II FMR is noted on the left foot and Type I FMR on the right foot. This patient's postoperative course permitted day-1 weightbearing as tolerated in surgical shoes for 6 weeks, then transitioned into stable sneakers.

with MI (varying subcapital osteotomy) and open treatment (Scarf, Lapidus or big toe arthrodesis) involving 143 publications concluded that "MI did not show worse outcomes or safety concerns."[74]

As MIBS becomes more prevalent, more outcome focused research studies will continue to emerge making comparative meta-analysis more meaningful. Moreover, the challenge of any MIBS study will be to differentiate between the variations between generations, osteotomy type, fixation type, number of screws, bunion size, and surgeon experience influences.

DISCUSSION

While MIBS is indeed a game-changing surgical solution for hallux valgus, its widespread adoption has been snail's pace slow.[1] Foot and ankle surgeons have been cautious to rapidly adopt this new version MIBS because the technique and fixation methods do not follow classic bunion surgery AO principles. Moreover, the visual appearance of bony segments in discontinuity stabilized by bridging screws traversing

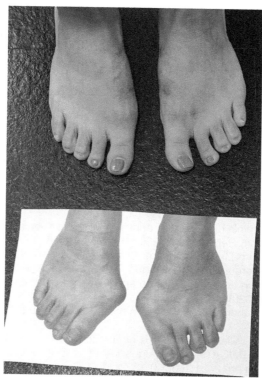

Fig. 13. Clinical result of patient in **Fig. 11** who underwent same day bilateral single screw construct and stabilizing osteotomy MIBS. These results are spectacular considering the severity of the deformities that were able to be treated with through tiny incisions, a single screw in each foot and healing by natural bone regeneration (rather than force fusion). Moreover, this patient was permitted a functional walking recovery without casts or crutches. The clinical end-result demonstrates how revolutionary MIBS is and a testament as to why it is the end-all be-all of bunion surgery.

a large osseous defect is disconcerting to the untrained eye. Now that studies have emerged demonstrating that the bones heal (FMR classification) and results/outcomes are at least consistent if not better than traditional bunion surgery, surgeons are rapidly flocking to receive training.

As far as being an ideal bunionectomy procedure, MIBS seems to properly address all the pain points of recovery, cosmesis, complications, and outcomes. The laparoscopic-like procedure allows structural osseous realignment of bunions of all sizes without sacrificing one natural-born joint anatomy (no-fusion) with a walking recovery. Seems that the negative perception of bunion surgery will fade, as will the need for so many procedures, making MIBS likely the most common bunion procedure performed and "end-all be-all" bunion repair method.

CLINICS CARE POINTS

- MIBS is performed as fluoroscopic guided using rotary burs and advanced screw technology.
- Various subcapital osteotomies have been described (transverse, chevron, and Transveron™).
- Realignment involves shifting bones into discontinuity with a fixation construct that spans an osseous defect that heals via callus formation (a.k.a., first metatarsal regeneration—FMR).

- A 1-screw or 2-screw MIBS construct can be used, depending on osteotomy configuration and screw/construct stability.
- MIBS is being rapidly adopted and quickly becoming the new gold standard surgical bunion method.

DISCLOSURE

Dr N. Blitz is the CEO of Voom Medical Devices Inc and receives compensation for this role.

REFERENCES

1. Blitz NM. New minimally invasive bunion surgery: easier said than done. Foot Ankle Surg: techn. Rep Cases 2023;3(4):2023-100288.
2. Vernois J, Redfern D. Percutaneous Chevron; the union of classic stable fixed approach and percutaneous technique. Fuß Sprunggelenk 2013;11:70–5.
3. Redfern D, Vernois J, Legré BP. Percutaneous surgery of the forefoot. Clin Podiatr Med Surg 2015;32(3):291–332.
4. Blitz NM. Game-changing new modern minimally invasive surgery. Foot Ankle Q 2020;31:181–91.
5. Lewis TL, Ray R, Miller G, et al. Third-generation minimally invasive chevron and Akin osteotomies (MICA) in hallux valgus surgery: two-year follow-up of 292 cases. J Bone Joint Surg Am 2021;103(13):1203–11.
6. Blitz NM. Current concepts in minimally invasive bunion surgery. Podiatry Today 2019;32(2).
7. Toepfer A, Strässle M. The percutaneous learning curve of 3rd generation minimally-invasive Chevron and Akin osteotomy (MICA). Foot Ankle Surg 2022; 28(8):1389–98.
8. Baumann AN, Walley KC, Anastasio AT, et al. Learning curve associated with minimally invasive surgery for hallux valgus: a systematic review. Foot Ankle Surg 2023;29(8):560–5.
9. Blitz NM, Grecea B, Wong DT, et al. Defining the cortical Purchase zone in new minimally invasive bunion surgery. A retrospective study of 638 cases. J Min Invasive Bunion Surg 2024;1:92777.
10. Lu J, Zhao H, Liang X, et al. Comparison of minimally invasive and traditionally open surgeries in correction of hallux valgus: a meta-analysis. J Foot Ankle Surg 2020;59(4):801–6.
11. Blitz NM, Wong DT, Grecea B, et al. Characterization of first metatarsal regeneration after a new modern minimally invasive bunion surgery. A retrospective radiographic review of 172 cases. J Min Invasive Bunion Surg 2024;1:92756.
12. Trnka HJ. Osteotomies for hallux valgus correction. Foot Ankle Clin 2005;10(1): 15–33.
13. Sorensen MD, Gradisek B, Cottom JM. Metatarsus primus varus correction. Clin Podiatr Med Surg 2015;32(3):355–74.
14. Wanivenhaus A, Bock P, Gruber F, et al. Deformitätsassoziierte Behandlung des Hallux-valgus-Komplexes [Deformity-associated treatment of the hallux valgus complex]. Orthopä 2009;38(11):1117–26. German.
15. Weil L Jr, Bowen M. Scarf osteotomy for correction of hallux abducto valgus deformity. Clin Podiatr Med Surg 2014;31(2):233–46.

16. Gerbert J. Textbook of bunion surgery. United States: Data Trace Publishing Company; 2012.

17. Valgus H. Forefoot surgery. United Kingdom: Churchill Livingstone; 1994.

18. Dayton P, Kauwe M, Feilmeier M. Is our current paradigm for evaluation and management of the bunion deformity flawed? A discussion of procedure philosophy relative to anatomy. J Foot Ankle Surg 2015;54(1):102–11.

19. Blitz NM. Preface: the surgical playbook. Clin Podiatr Med Surg 2010;27(1): xvii–xviii.

20. Sammarco GJ, Idusuyi OB. Complications after surgery of the hallux. Clin Orthop Relat Res 2001;391:59–71.

21. Thompson FM. Complications of hallux valgus surgery and salvage. Orthopedics 1990;13(9):1059–67.

22. Belczyk R, Stapleton JJ, Grossman JP, et al. Complications and revisional hallux valgus surgery. Clin Podiatr Med Surg 2009;26(3):475–84. Table of Contents.

23. Barg A, Harmer JR, Presson AP, et al. Unfavorable outcomes following surgical treatment of hallux valgus deformity: a systematic literature review. J Bone Joint Surg Am 2018;100(18):1563–73.

24. Ezzatvar Y, López-Bueno L, Fuentes-Aparicio L, et al. Prevalence and predisposing factors for recurrence after hallux valgus surgery: a systematic review and meta-analysis. J Clin Med 2021;10(24):5753.

25. AlMeshari A, AlShehri Y, Anderson L, et al. Inconsistency in the reporting terminology of adverse events and complications in hallux valgus reconstruction: a systematic review. Foot Ankle Spec 2024;24:19386400241256215. https://doi.org/10.1177/19386400241256215.

26. Waehner M, Klos K, Polzer H, et al. Lapidus arthrodesis for correction of hallux valgus deformity: a systematic review and meta-analysis. Foot Ankle Spec 2024;19386400241233832. https://doi.org/10.1177/19386400241233832.

27. McBride ED. A conservative operation for bunions. 1928. J Bone Joint Surg Am 2002;84(11):2101.

28. Yucel I, Tenekecioglu Y, Ogut T, et al. Treatment of hallux valgus by modified McBride procedure: a 6-year follow-up. J Orthop Traumatol 2010;11(2):89–97.

29. Blitz NM. Current concepts in medial column hypermobility. Podiatry Today 2005;18(6).

30. Gill LH. Distal osteotomy for bunionectomy and hallux valgus correction. Foot Ankle Clin 2001;6(3):433–53.

31. Piccora RN. The Austin bunionectomy: then and now. Clin Podiatr Med Surg 1989;6(1):179–96.

32. Clancy JT, Berlin SJ, Giordano ML, et al. Modified Austin bunionectomy with single screw fixation: a comparison study. J Foot Surg 1989;28(4):284–9.

33. Boggs SI, Selner AJ, Roth IE, et al. Tricorrectional bunionectomy with AO screw fixation. J Foot Surg 1989;28(3):185–90.

34. Goforth WP, Martin JE. Eighteen-month retrospective study of Austin bunionectomy using single screw fixation. J Foot Ankle Surg 1993;32(1):69–74.

35. Hill RS, Marek LJ. Modification of the Kalish osteotomy to correct the proximal articular set angle. J Am Podiatr Med Assoc 1990;80(8):424–8.

36. Gerbert J. Complications of the austin-type bunionectomy. J Foot Surg 1978; 17(1):1–6.

37. Trnka HJ, Hofmann S, Salzer M, et al. Clinical and radiological results after Austin bunionectomy for treatment of hallux valgus. Arch Orthop Trauma Surg 1996; 115(3–4):171–5.

38. Coetzee JC. Scarf osteotomy for hallux valgus repair: the dark side. Foot Ankle Int 2003;24(1):29–33.
39. Clemente P, Mariscal G, Barrios C. Distal chevron osteotomy versus different operative procedures for hallux valgus correction: a meta-analysis. J Orthop Surg Res 2022;17:80.
40. Nigro JS, Greger GM, Catanzariti AR. Closing base wedge osteotomy. J Foot Surg 1991;30(5):494–505.
41. Morris J, Ryan M. First metatarsal base osteotomies for hallux abducto valgus deformities. Clin Podiatr Med Surg 2014;31(2):247–63.
42. Blitz NM. The versatility of the Lapidus arthrodesis. Clin Podiatr Med Surg 2009; 26(3):427–41.
43. Blitz NM, Lee T, Williams K, et al. Early weight bearing after modified lapidus arthodesis: a multicenter review of 80 cases. J Foot Ankle Surg 2010;49(4):357–62.
44. Blitz NM. Early weightbearing of the lapidus: is it possible? Podiatry Today 2004;17(8).
45. Dujela MD, Langan T, Cottom JM, et al. Lapidus arthrodesis. Clin Podiatr Med Surg 2022;39(2):187–206.
46. King CM, Castellucci-Garza FM. The lapidus bunionectomy revolution: current concepts and considerations. Clin Podiatr Med Surg 2024;41(1):43–58.
47. Dayton P, Feilmeier M, Kauwe M, et al. Relationship of frontal plane rotation of first metatarsal to proximal articular set angle and hallux alignment in patients undergoing tarsometatarsal arthrodesis for hallux abducto valgus: a case series and critical review of the literature. J Foot Ankle Surg 2013;52(3):348–54.
48. Wang B, Manchanda K, Lalli T, et al. Identifying risk factors for nonunion of the modified lapidus procedure for the correction of hallux valgus. J Foot Ankle Surg 2022;61(5):1001–6.
49. Patel S, Ford LA, Etcheverry J, et al. Modified lapidus arthrodesis: rate of nonunion in 227 cases. J Foot Ankle Surg 2004;43(1):37–42.
50. Buddecke DE Jr, Reese ER, Prusa RD. Revision of malaligned lapidus and nonunited lapidus. Clin Podiatr Med Surg 2020;37(3):505–20.
51. McKean RM, Bergin PF, Watson G, et al. Radiographic evaluation of intermetatarsal angle correction following first MTP joint arthrodesis for severe hallux valgus. Foot Ankle Int 2016;37(11):1183–6.
52. Rippstein PF, Park YU, Naal FD. Combination of first metatarsophalangeal joint arthrodesis and proximal correction for severe hallux valgus deformity. Foot Ankle Int 2012;33(5):400–5.
53. Kunovsky R, Kocis J, Navrat T, et al. Lapidus arthrodesis in combination with arthrodesis of the first metatarsophalangeal joint-biomechanical cadaver study comparing two methods of fixation. Biomed Pap Med Fac Univ Palacky Olomouc Czech Repub 2022;166(3):334–42.
54. Trnka HJ. Percutaneous, MIS and open hallux valgus surgery. EFORT Open Rev 2021;6(6):432–8.
55. Isham SA. The Reverdin-Isham procedure for the correction of hallux abducto valgus. A distal metatarsal osteotomy procedure. Clin Podiatr Med Surg 1991; 8(1):81–94.
56. Bösch P, Wanke S, Legenstein R. Hallux valgus correction by the method of Bösch: a new technique with a seven-to-ten-year follow-up. Foot Ankle Clin 2000;5(3):485–98, v-vi.
57. Giannini S, Faldini C, Vannini F, et al. The minimally invasive osteotomy "S.E.R.I." (simple, effective, rapid, inexpensive) for correction of bunionette deformity. Foot Ankle Int 2008;29(3):282–6.

58. Lewis TL, Lau B, Alkhalfan Y, et al. Fourth-generation minimally invasive hallux valgus surgery with metaphyseal extra-articular transverse and Akin osteotomy (META): 12 Month clinical and radiologic results. Foot Ankle Int 2023;44(3):178–91.

59. Ferreira GF, Nunes GA, Dorado DS, et al. Correction of first metatarsal pronation in metaphyseal extra-articular transverse osteotomy for hallux valgus correction. Foot & Ankle Orthopaedics 2023;8(3). https://doi.org/10.1177/24730114231198527.

60. Voom Medical Devices, Co. Revcon minimally invasive screw system surgical technique. Available at: https://www.voommedicaldevices.com/files/2023_Voom_OpTech_Complete_Digital_01.pdf.

61. Wong DT. A new paradigm for failed bunions with minimally invasive methods. Clin Podiatr Med Surg 2025;42(1):102–16.

62. Blitz NM, Wong DT, Baskin ES. Patterns of metatarsal explosion after new modern minimally invasive bunion surgery. A retrospective review and case series of 16 feet. J Min Invasive Bunion Surg 2024;1:92774.

63. Di Nucci KA. The unfamiliar complications of minimally invasive foot surgery. Clin Podiatr Med Surg 2025;42(1):117–38.

64. AOFAS Position Statement, Minimally invasive surgery (MIS) for hallux valgus (HV) deformity, American Orthopedic Foot & Ankle Society, 2024.

65. Lewis TL, Ray R, Robinson P, et al. Percutaneous chevron and Akin (PECA) osteotomies for severe hallux valgus deformity with mean 3-year follow-up. Foot Ankle Int 2021;42(10):1231–40.

66. Neufeld SK, Dean D, Hussaini S. Outcomes and surgical strategies of minimally invasive chevron/akin procedures. Foot Ankle Int 2021;42(6):676–88.

67. Holme TJ, Sivaloganathan SS, Patel B, et al. Third-generation minimally invasive chevron Akin osteotomy for hallux valgus. Foot Ankle Int 2020;41(1):50–6.

68. Anciano Granadillo VJ, Werner BC, Moran TE, et al. Perioperative opioid analgesics and hallux valgus correction surgery: trends, risk factors for prolonged use and complications. J Foot Ankle Surg 2022;61(6):1152–7.

69. Caolo KC, Marion C, Paugh R, et al. Prescribing fewer opioid pills to hallux valgus patients undergoing minimally invasive bunion correction: a prospective comparative study. Foot Ankle Orthop 2022;7(1):2473011421S00127. https://doi.org/10.1177/2473011421S00127.

70. Mikhail CM, Markowitz J, Di Lenarda L, et al. Clinical and radiographic outcomes of percutaneous chevron-akin osteotomies for the correction of hallux valgus deformity. Foot Ankle Int 2022;43(1):32–41.

71. Roukis TS. Percutaneous and minimum incision metatarsal osteotomies: a systematic review. J Foot Ankle Surg 2009;48(3):380–7.

72. Malagelada F, Sahirad C, Dalmau-Pastor M, et al. Minimally invasive surgery for hallux valgus: a systematic review of current surgical techniques. Int Orthop 2019;43(3):625–37.

73. Ji L, Wang K, Ding S, et al. Minimally invasive vs. Open surgery for hallux valgus: a meta-analysis. Front Surg 2022;9:843410.

74. Nair A, Bence M, Saleem J, et al. A systematic review of open and minimally invasive surgery for treating recurrent hallux valgus. Surg J (N Y) 2022;8(4):e350–6.

Management of Hammer Toe Deformities Using Percutaneous Surgical Techniques

Adam Reaney, BSc (Hons), MRCPod, LLCM, ARSM[a],
Togay Koç, MBBS, MSc, FRCS (Tr & Orth)[b],
Thomas L. Lewis, MBChB (Hons), BSc (Hons), FRCS (Tr & Orth), MFSTEd[c],
David Gordon, MB ChB, MRCS, MD, FRCS (Tr & Orth)[d,*]

KEYWORDS

- Percutaneous surgery • Minimally invasive surgery • Hammer toe

KEY POINTS

- Hammer toe deformity is a prevalent condition, which presents significant discomfort, reduces mobility, and reduces patient quality of life.
- Thorough anatomic knowledge and biomechanic understanding of the lesser metatarsophalangeal joint complex is imperative for accurate diagnosis and management of hammer toe deformity.
- Conservative measures can provide short-term symptom relief, but surgical correction is required for long-term curative treatment of the pathology.
- Minimally invasive surgery procedures incorporating soft tissue releases and osteotomies offer effective long-term correction with minimal tissue trauma.

INTRODUCTION

Hammer toe deformity is frequently defined as a toe with flexion of the proximal interphalangeal joint (PIPJ), metatarsophalangeal joint (MTPJ) extension, with or without distal interphalangeal joint (DIPJ) involvement[1] (**Fig. 1**). Hammer toe may initially present as a flexible deformity, but as it progresses it may become more rigid.

Hammer toe deformities are present in one-third of the population, thus, accounting for a high proportion of visits to foot and ankle clinics.[2] Although genetics play a role in its pathophysiology, risk factors for the condition include: hallux valgus deformity, inflammatory arthropathies, advanced age, trauma, and neuromuscular conditions.[3] This may cause discomfort or pain in footwear due to rubbing, impacting, walking, and activities.

[a] Cardiff University School of Medicine, Cardiff, UK; [b] University Hospital Southampton NHS Foundation Trust, Southampton, UK; [c] King's College Hospital NHS Foundation NHS Trust, London, UK; [d] The London Clinic, 20 Devonshire Place, Marylebone, London W1G 6BW, UK
* Corresponding author.
E-mail address: research@davidgordonortho.com

Clin Podiatr Med Surg 42 (2025) 33–46
https://doi.org/10.1016/j.cpm.2024.06.001
podiatric.theclinics.com
0891-8422/25/Crown Copyright © 2024 Published by Elsevier Inc. All rights are reserved, including those for text and data mining, AI training, and similar technologies.

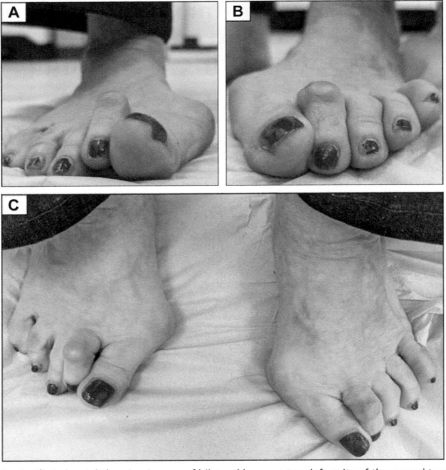

Fig. 1. Clinical weightbearing images of bilateral hammer toe deformity of the second toes in the clinical setting of concomitant hallux valgus. The marked proximal interphalangeal joint flexion and associated dorsal callosities in evident in all views (*A*) Right Foot, (*B*) Left Foot, (*C*) Top Down view.

There is significant literature discussing hammer toe correction via open techniques;[4,5] however, there is a paucity of literature discussing minimally invasive or percutaneous techniques to treat this pathology.[3] Mateen and colleagues performed a comparative study and found the minimally invasive surgery (MIS) hammer toe procedure provides similar results to the open procedure with an earlier return to normal footwear (2 weeks in MIS vs 6 weeks in open).[3] This article aims to review hammer toe deformity and specifically, the MIS options used to treat the condition.

RELEVANT ANATOMY

The anatomy of the plantar plate, extensor apparatus, and static and dynamic stabilizers of the MTPJ are the keys to maintaining structure, function, and alignment. Pathology affecting these structures can lead to an imbalance of forces and lead to development of deformity.

Plantar Plate of the lesser Metatarsophalangeal Joint's

The plantar plate is a broad fibrocartilaginous ribbon-like disc structure composed predominantly of Type 1 Collagen (75%), which acts as the main static stabilizer of lesser MTPJ's. It has a rectangular to trapezoidal shape with a range in thickness, length and width between; 2 to 5 mm, 16 to 23 mm, and 8 to 13 mm, respectively.[6] It originates from the periosteum of the distal end of the metatarsal shaft and inserts to the plantar aspect of the proximal phalanx. The plantar plate inserts in 2 major portions- the medial and lateral bundles, which form a 'socket' for the metatarsal head to slide in during dorsiflexion and plantarflexion[7] (**Fig. 2**). The plantar surface is smooth and grooved at its peripheries providing a gliding plane for the flexor tendons.[7,8] The plantar plate is thickest at its mid-portion and thinnest at its metatarsal origin, whilst at the phalangeal insertion, its borders are thicker than its central section.[7]

The majority of the plantar plate fibers run longitudinally in line with the plantar fascia allowing the plantar plate to withstand increased tensile loads (required for the windlass mechanism).

The plantar plate is the main static stabilizer of the lesser MTPJ's and also acts as the insertion point for other static stabilizers including the collateral ligaments and the deep transverse intermetatarsal metatarsal ligament (IML). These structures compose a secure 'box like' structure, which aid static stabilization of the lesser MTPJ's.[9]

STATIC STABILISERS OF THE LESSER METATARSOPHALANGEAL JOINT'S

The collateral ligaments provide significant attachment of the plate to the metatarsal head[7] and the IML attaches to the medial and lateral aspects of the plantar plate.[8,10]

DYNAMIC STABILISERS OF THE LESSER METATARSOPHALANGEAL JOINT'S

These include the flexor and extensor apparatus consisting of extensor digitorum longus (EDL) and extensor digitorum brevis (EDB), which lie dorsally, and flexor digitorum longus (FDL) and flexor digitorum brevis (FDB) which lie plantarly.[9] The FDL and FDB reside within their sheath plantar to the plantar plate.[8,10] Additionally, four lumbrical muscles originate

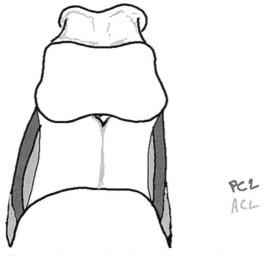

Fig. 2. A schematic showing the medial and lateral bundles of the plantar plate inserting into the plantar aspect of the proximal phalanx.

from the medial border of FDL tendons and insert into the medial side of the proximal phalanx on the plantar surface and insert into the distal plantar aspect of the plantar plate.[8,10]

HAMMER TOE DEFORMITY ETIOLOGY

Specific causes of hammer toe deformity include: hallux valgus, a short first metatarsal (index minus), soft-tissue lesions affecting the extensors or flexors, and central or peripheral neurologic disease (resulting in intrinsic and extrinsic muscle imbalance). Furthermore, joint destruction by rheumatoid or osteoarthritis and post trauma malunion are also common etiologies.[11] It is widely accepted that muscular imbalance between strong extrinsic and weak intrinsic musculature play a pivotal role in pathophysiology.[12] Plantar plate attenuation or injury, leading to proximal phalanx subluxation and MTPJ extension also plays a role.[1,13]

The primary etiology of hammer toe deformity is a muscular imbalance between strong extrinsic muscles and weak intrinsic muscles. When the proximal phalanx is in neutral position, the EDL extends the PIPJ and DIPJ and FDL flexes the MTPJ. However, muscular imbalance causing proximal phalanx extension, results in EDL losing its mechanical advantage, resulting in PIPJ and DIPJ flexion from the unopposed long flexor. The lumbricals and interossei are the only counteracting extensors of the IPJ's, but these are weak, easily overpowered by stronger extrinsic muscles and are off axis, resulting in MTPJ extension. Furthermore, the lesser MTPJ complex is mainly passively stabilised in the sagittal plane by the plantar plate, collateral ligaments, and joint capsule, which limit MTPJ dorsiflexion during gait. As the deformity progresses, the plantar plate attenuates and leads to subluxation of the proximal phalanx dorsally on the metatarsal head.[10] Subsequently, pulling the metatarsal fat pad distally and depressing the metatarsal head plantarly,[1] leading to further proximal phalanx hyperextension, which is key to its pathophysiology.[14]

Furthermore, Dhukaram and colleagues[13] found that narrow, short footwear with a high heel forces the MTPJ into hyperextension and the PIPJ into flexion, which can cause stretching and failure of the plantar plate and thus, is often implicated in the causation of the deformity.[5]

Hallux valgus is often associated with hammer toe deformity and often contributes toward its etiology, due to its resulting shortening of the first ray, which slackens the plantar fascia and weakens the windlass effect on the great toe. Therefore, increasing the strain on the lesser toes, resulting in the eventual attenuation and destruction of their supporting structures.[5]

Diagnosis

An accurate diagnosis is crucial to ensure effective and efficient management of the hammer toe deformity. The diagnosis should not only confirm the presence of the deformity, but also stage the severity of the deformity, which in turn informs the management options. Clinical examination and imaging should be used to inform conservative management or surgical planning.

Clinical examination

A thorough clinical examination is imperative to ascertain the degree of deformity and to aid the correct selection of surgical management.

Firstly, the clinician should observe the foot in weight-bearing and non-weight-bearing, taking note of other deformities for example, claw toe, mallet toe, or hallux valgus, in addition to callosities on the dorsal DIPJ, PIPJ or plantar MTPJ.

The level of flexibility and rigidity of the DIPJ, PIPJ, and MTPJ should be examined by physical movement of the joints as these inform the method of treatment. The ability to passively correct the deformity is a flexible deformity, whilst the inability to passively correct it, is a rigid deformity. Flexor tendon tightness can be assessed by moving the ankle from dorsiflexion to plantarflexion. A flexible hammer toe deformity will correct itself as the ankle is brought into plantarflexion. Palpation of the plantar forefoot at the base of involved toes should be performed to identify MTPJ localized tenderness or interdigital neuromas.[4]

Metatarsophalangeal joint instability

Instability of the MTPJ may coexist with a hammer toe deformity and assessing this by Lachman's test to ascertain the integrity of the plantar plate must be performed when considering hammer toe correction. To perform Lachman's test; whilst the patient is non-weight-bearing, the clinician holds the metatarsal head between their thumb and index finger and, with the other hand, moves the toe dorsally. A positive Lachman's test is indicative of toe subluxation.[15] Lachman's test findings aid assessment of MTPJ stability (**Table 1**).

Furthermore, the clinician should also observe the patient's gait to assess; the deformity during gait, walking aid usage, orthotic therapy usage, and ascertain the neurologic status of the foot during gait.[5] Ankle range-of-motion should also be assessed to ascertain if ankle equinus is contributing toward the deformity, as this would influence surgical management.

Imaging

Weight-bearing anteroposterior and lateral radiographs aid hammer toe diagnosis by assessing congruency of the lesser MTPJs, degree of flexion, and extension at the MTPJ, PIPJ, and DIPJ. Radiographs also enable evaluation of the metatarsal parabola, a short first metatarsal (index minus), joint condition, and associated pathologies such as hallux valgus and crossover deformity.[9]

Diagnostic ultrasound is a common modality used to image the plantar plate and enables the clinician to stress the joint (eg, perform a drawer test) with direct visualization of the structures during imaging.[16] Evidence of MTPJ synovitis and other arthritides can also be identified. Ultrasound is accessible and inexpensive but operator dependent.

Table 1
MTPJ condition and associated clinical findings indicative of positive or negative Lachman's test.

MTPJ Condition	Lachman Test	Clinical Finding
Stable	Negative	MTPJ moves noramally in the sagittal plane
Unstable	Positive	MTPJ moves abnoramally in the sagittal plane
Subluxable	Positive	MTPJ moves abnoramally in the sagittal plane but not dislocatable
Dislocatable	Positive	MTPJ is dislocatable in the sagittal plane or is dislocated on weight-bearing but fully reducible with manual reduction (however, may not remain reduced on weight-bearing)
Fixed (irreducible) dislocation	N/A	MTPJ cannot be reduced manually to anatomically normal

Abbreviation: MTPJ, metatarsophalangeal joint.

With 95% sensitivity and 100% specificity, MRI has become the most useful imaging technique to assess plantar plate integrity. On MRI, areas of hyperintense T2 signal around the plantar plate's distal attachment, joint effusion, and pericapsular fibrosis are all features of plantar plate injury[17] (**Fig. 3**).

A systematic review and meta-analysis by Albright and colleagues found that MRI was superior to ultrasound to diagnose plantar plate pathologies; however, they found ultrasound had a higher sensitivity than MRI. A strength of MRI is its ability to evaluate the integrity of associated structures such as the flexors, extensors, and collateral and suspensory ligaments, in addition to identifying pathologies such as Morton's neuroma, capsulitis, bone marrow oedema and osteochondral lesions.[18]

Management

Conservative management

Footwear modifications or changes such as adopting a shoe with a wide and deep toe box and low heel along with orthotic therapy can also help manage the deformity.[19]

When the deformity is flexible and fully correctable, adhesive taping and splinting (Budin splint, branded hammer toe splints) may be used to maintain the MTPJ and PIPJs in neutral positions. This may provide relief and reduce the pressure on the dorsal aspect of the digit.

Silicone moulded toe props can be used to reduce peak pressure and pressure-time on the apex of the digits with flexible and rigid hammer toe toe deformities. This reduction in peak pressure on the skin also reduces the risk of ulceration, especially if there is a neuropathic component to the pathology. Furthermore, it reduces the likelihood of corn development, thus, reducing pain on walking, subsequently reducing fall risk.[20] Regular debridement of associated hyperkeratosis will reduce peak pressure and reduce ulceration risk.[21]

It is accepted that conservative treatment for hammer toe is not a curative measure, but simply a management of the symptoms of hammer toe deformity. For long-term term curative treatment, surgical intervention may be required.

Surgical Management

(Minimally invasive surgical procedures). A number of MIS surgical procedures can be utilized to correct the hammer toe deformity, either in isolation or in combination.

1. PIPJ FDB release
2. Dorsal PIPJ skin excision and suturing (DSES)

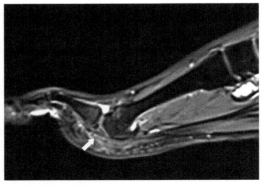

Fig. 3. A T2 MRI scan showing hyperintense signal at the second metatarsophalangeal joint (MTPJ) complex indicative of plantar plate rupture (*arrow*).

3. Proximal phalangeal (P1) basal osteotomy
4. PIPJ fusion with intramedullary screw
5. Distal metaphyseal metatarsal osteotomy (DMMO)
6. MTPJ soft tissue procedures (capsular release, tenotomy, and tendon lengthening)

The procedure choice or combination will depend on the flexibility of the PIPJ deformity and the stability of the MTPJ.

The following flow chart provides a treatment algorithm for the surgical management of the hammer toe deformity (**Fig. 4**).

FLEXIBILITY OF THE PROXIMAL INTERPHALANGEAL JOINT DEFORMITY
The Flexibility of the Proximal Interphalangeal Joint (PIPJ) is Assessed and Falls into Three Categories, Listed Below:

Fully flexible
PIPJ held in a flexed position but can achieve full extension passively. If the PIPJ achieves full extension on manual plantar flexion pressure, at the P1 base, then a P1 basal osteotomy (combined if needed with DSES) may be utilized.

Partly flexible
Some passive PIPJ extension can be achieved although not full extension. An FDB release will convert the deformity to a flexible deformity to allow treatment as a fully flexible deformity.

Fixed Deformity
No passive PIPJ extension can be achieved (i.e., fixed flexion). Due to the higher risk of recurrence, the author prefers to perform a FDB release, a percutaneous PIPJ fusion with an intramedullary screw, in combination with a P1 basal osteotomy to correct any residual deformity.

STABILITY OF THE METATARSOPHALANGEAL JOINT

A pain free and stable MTPJ, with an associated hammer toe deformity, does not require further procedures to the MTPJ. However, if MTPJ instability is identified, or

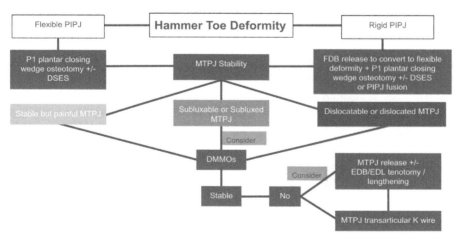

Fig. 4. A flow chart illustrating a treatment algorithm for the surgical management of hammer toe deformity.

a painful but stable MTPJ exists, then further MIS procedures should be utilized according to the degree of instability.

STABLE BUT PAINFUL

Dorsal or plantar MTPJ pain may be resolved by shortening and elevating the metatarsal head with a distal metatarsal osteotomy distal metaphyseal metatarsal osteotomy (DMMO). It is recommended to perform adjacent metatarsal DMMOs to reduce the risk of a transfer lesion, where new plantar pain occurs post operatively. For a second DMMO planned, include a third DMMO, for a third DMMO planned, include a second and fourth DMMO.

SUBLUXABLE OR SUBLUXED

Depending on the degree of subluxation, which can be achieved, it is clinical judgment whether a metatarsal osteotomy is required. In mild to moderate subluxation, a metatarsal osteotomy may not be needed; however, in more significant subluxation, a DMMO should be considered.

DISLOCATABLE

Significant plantar plate attenuation has occurred, therefore, a DMMO is recommended. An alternative to this, is an open plantar plate repair; however, the senior author tends to avoid this procedure due to the high risk of stiffness and floating toe.

FIXED (IRREDUCIBLE) DISLOCATION

This situation presents a challenging problem for the surgeon. However, a DMMO often allows the MTPJ to be reduced; however, may remain unstable intraoperatively despite this. A trans-articular K-wire (KW) can be used temporarily for 6 weeks to induce some stiffness and therefore, stability in the joint. The KW is inserted through the tip of the toe penetrating the DIPJ, PIPJ, MTPJ, and into the intramedullary canal of the metatarsal, to stop at the tarsoometatarsal joint. A dorsal MTPJ percutaneous release may also be used, alongside an extensor tendon Z lengthening.

SURGICAL TECHNIQUE OPTIONS
Proximal Interphalangeal Joint Flexor Digitorum Brevis Release

A Beaver blade is inserted either medially or laterally, through the toe skin, at the level of the PIPJ, aiming to skirt the distal plantar P1 condyles. The PIPJ is held in 30° of flexion. Keeping the blade pointing distally (not plantar, so avoiding the FDL), the blade is carefully mobilized in an oscillating fashion, in a distal direction, on bone, to release the plantar plate and the medial and lateral FBD slips. An incomplete release (correction of PIPJ flexion) is preferred, as manual hyperextension of the PIPJ is a safer method to complete the release than multiple attempts with the Beaver blade. Wounds are irrigated, and then closed with adhesive strips.

Dorsal Proximal Interphalangeal Joint Skin Excision and Suturing

If further extension is desired, a dorsal PIPJ skin ellipse is excised and closed with sutures, enough to bring the PIPJ to neutral extension.

Proximal Phalangeal Basal Osteotomy

The plantar metatarsal head is palpated with the non-dominant thumb and a Beaver blade is inserted through skin only, just distal to this point. A 2 mm wide x 8 mm long Shannon burr is inserted through the incision aiming toward the P1 base through the flexor tendons. Once bone is felt, the burr is advanced through the planter cortex of the P1, until it abuts but does not go through the dorsal cortex. A radiograph image confirms the position of the burr, ensuring it is not in the MTPJ, not in the P1 diaphysis but at the P1 metaphyseal diaphyseal junction and central. The burr is repositioned as necessary.

A plantar wedge is then removed keeping the dorsal cortex intact, by sweeping the burr both medially and laterally. The toe is then pushed into plantar flexion, closing the osteotomy. A click may be heard as the dorsal cortex breaks but this is not a concern (**Fig. 5**). Simulated weight bearing is performed to assess the degree of toe correction and ideally the corrected toe ought to be lower than the other adjacent, normal toes. Wounds are irrigated, then closed with adhesive strips.

Alternatively, through-and-through P1 osteotomies could be performed and oriented/angulated to correct deformity and realign the digit, particularly for more complex digital deformities (i.e., crossover toes) (**Fig. 6**).

Proximal Interphalangeal Joint Fusion with Intrameduallary Screw

PIPJ fusion is performed before any P1 basal osteotomy or distal metatarsal osteotomy, as bony stability is required.

A PIPJ FDB release is performed, and utilising the same incision, a 2 mm wide x 8 mm long Shannon burr is inserted into the PIPJ. A radiograph image confirms the burr is perpendicular to the long axis of the P1. The cartilage of P1 is then removed, utilizing radiographs to ensure bone removal remains perpendicular to the long axis of P1. Using a sponge holder to grasp the tip of the toe to distract the excised PIPJ, a radiograph can be taken to assess adequacy of resection.

A 3 mm incision is made at the tip of the toe with a Beaver blade and a 0.9 KW advanced intramedullary to the base of P1. Dorso-plantar and lateral radiographs are taken to confirm the KW position. The KW is measured, ensuring the desired screw length is from the distal margin of P2, to circa 3 mm proximal to the P1 diaphysis. This ensures enough space is available to perform a basal P1 osteotomy without encroaching on the tip of the screw.

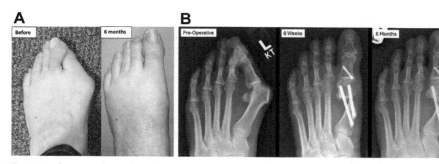

Fig. 5. Before & after clinical image and radiographs demonstrating minimally invasive bunion and minimally invasive hammer toe correction of the second toe. The bunion deformity was corrected by a percutaneous distal first metatarsal fixation with dual metatarsal screws, resolving the underriding hallux. The second toe was corrected through P1 osteotomy.

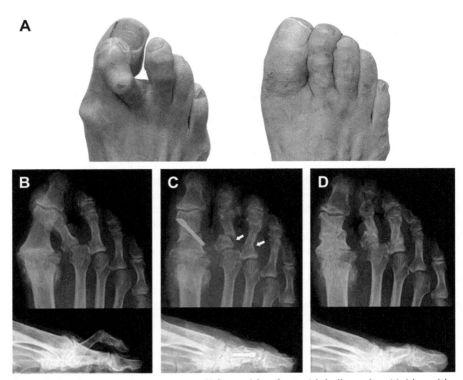

Fig. 6. Series demonstrating treatment disfigured forefoot with hallux valgus/rigidus with a crossover 2nd toe and hammer toe of the 3rd toe. (*A*) Clinical images before and after correct demonstrate the severity of the deformity and return of the toes to the rectus position. (*B*) Pre-operative radiographs the subluxation of the 2nd and 3rd MTPJ's and flexion contracture at the PIPJ. Hallux abduction secondary to 1st MTPJ arthrosis was evident. (*C*) Postoperative image illustrating P1 osteotomies of the 2nd and 3rd toes (arrows). A middle phalanx osteotomy was performed on the 2nd toe along with a capsular MPTJ release with extensor tenotomy. Percutaneous cheilectomy and Akin were performed to straighten the big toe. (*D*) Healed radiographic images demonstrate resolution of the crossover toes and healed osteotomies. (*Image courtesy of* Neal M. Blitz, DPM.)

Following drilling for the screw, the screw is inserted, ensuring the head of the screw passes beyond the DIPJ. It is helpful to hold the toe with a swab, maintaining correct rotational alignment and PIPJ compression. Dorso-plantar and lateral radiographs are taken to confirm the screw position. Simulated weight bearing is performed and a P1 basal osteotomy may now be performed if there is residual extension at the MTPJ (**Fig. 7**). Wounds are irrigated, then closed with adhesive strips.

Distal Metaphyseal Metatarsal Osteotomy

A detailed description of the surgical technique has been described by De Prado and colleagues[22] and Redfern and Vernois.[23] The surgeon stands at the end of the operating table, facing the soles of the feet. A 3 mm dorsal skin incision is made by the web space; its laterality to the metatarsal will be the same as the handedness of the surgeon regardless of the foot, for example, right-handed surgeon, the incision (and start position of the osteotomy) will be on the right hand side of the metatarsal.

Under fluoroscopic control, a 2 mm wide x 13 mm long Shannon burr is inserted through the incision, to rest on the metatarsal neck. The extra-articular osteotomy is

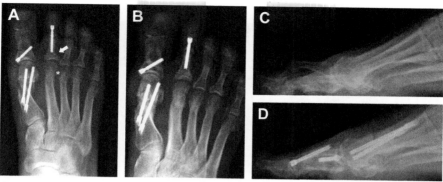

Fig. 7. Radiographs demonstrating rigid hammer toe correction of 2nd toe by proximal interphalangeal joint arthrodesis with PI plantarflexory base osteotomy and DMMO's of the 2nd and 3rd metatarsals. (*A*) Anteroposterior radiographs at 6 weeks. (*B*) Anteroposterior radiographs at 6 months demonstrating complete consolidation. (*C*) Preoperative lateral radiograph demonstrate the flexion contracture of the proximal interphalangeal joint along with dorsal extension contracture of the metatarsophalangeal joint. (*D*) Healed radiographs at 6 months reveal resolution on the hammer toe deformity.

made at 45° relative to the long axis of the metatarsal and in a dorsal-distal to proximal-plantar direction. The osteotomy is cut using a rotational movement of the burr hand piece, supinating the hand, pivoting about the incision. For a right DMMO (right-handed surgeon), the osteotomy is made progressively as follows: medial, plantar, lateral, and dorsal. Following completion, the osteotomy is gently stressed in a dorsal plantar and telescopic or axial fashion, to ensure complete mobility and shortening or position is confirmed fluoroscopically. Wounds are irrigated, and then closed with adhesive strips (**Fig. 8**).

Strapping is applied to maintain coronal and sagittal alignment and a stiff postoperative sandal applied. Two weeks of strict elevation but full weight-bearing is allowed, then transition to a normal, stiff-soled shoe at 4 weeks. Strapping is maintained for 6 weeks. Patients are advised of swelling and mild discomfort for up to 3 months.

Metatarsophalangeal Joint Soft Tissue Procedures

Several percutaneous soft tissue procedures may be added as required, to aid MTPJ correction. These are more likely required in fixed deformities and residual deformities following bony procedures. It is the senior author's preference to perform bony procedures first, and then assess the MTPJ position.

A dorsal capsular release (arthrolysis) is performed prior to considering extensor tendon surgery. It is performed under fluoroscopic control using a Beaver blade. An incision is made at level of MTPJ on the right side (if right-handed) and the joint entered, to release the dorsal capsule and the collaterals off the metatarsal head.

It is the senior author's preference to try and avoid extensor tenotomies or tendon lengthening, as disruption of these extrinsic forces after bony procedures can be detrimental to deformity correction. However, an EDB percutaneous tenotomy is performed 2 cm proximal to the MTPJ, where the tendon is lateral to EDL. Concurrent tenotomies of both EDB and EDL should be avoided, as this will lead to a 'dropped' toe that may catch on the ground.

An open Z lengthening of EDL may be performed following all other measures, if required.

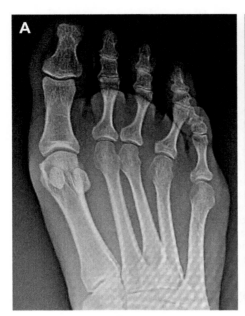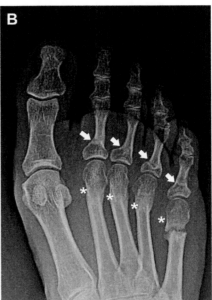

Fig. 8. Radiograph before and after hammer toe treatment of the 2nd, 3rd, 4th and 5th toes with P1 base osteotomies (arrows). Additionally, DMMO's (asterisks) were performed on corresponding metatarsals for the treatment of metatarsalgia. (*Image courtesy of* Eric S. Baskin, DPM.)

The following flow chart provides a treatment algorithm for the surgical management of hammer toe deformity (**Fig. 8**).

TOE STRAPPING

It is essential in the post-operative period, to maintain the toe in a corrected position. Various adhesive tapes can be utilized and the principles are to maintain the toe in a well-aligned and plantar-flexed position until bony union, which normally occurs by 6 weeks. Care is taken to protect with padding the dorsal basal skin of the toe during taping, as excessive plantar pressure can cause skin ulceration.

POST-OPERATIVE MOBILIZATION

Post-operative rehabilitation depends on whether any adjunctive procedures have been performed. If an isolated hammer toe correction has been undertaken, then it is recommended that the foot is elevated at the level of the waist, for 1 week. Full weight-bearing is possible immediately, in a flat rigid surgical sandal. It may be possible to transition from the surgical sandal into a normal stiff shoe after 2 weeks. If other more complex adjunctive procedures have been performed, then the rehabilitation will need to be tailored accordingly.

SUMMARY

In conclusion, hammer toe deformity presents significant discomfort and mobility issues for patients. While conservative measures offer temporary relief, surgical intervention, especially minimally invasive techniques, can provide long-term correction.

Understanding toe anatomy and biomechanics is crucial for accurate diagnosis and treatment planning. MIS procedures incorporating soft tissue releases and osteotomies offer effective correction with minimal tissue trauma. Post-operative care, including toe strapping and rehabilitation, is vital for optimal outcomes. Advanced techniques and ongoing research promise improved treatment efficacy, enhancing the quality of life for those affected by hammer toe deformity.

CLINICS CARE POINTS

- MRI has 95% sensitivity and 100% specificity when assessing plantar plate integrity,[17] although diagnostic ultrasound enables the joint to be stressed with direct visualization of the structures during imaging.[16]

- A systematic review and meta-analysis by Albright and colleagues found that MRI was superior to ultrasound to diagnose plantar plate pathologies.[18]

- Frequent intraoperative imaging should be used during initial burr placement, to ensure osteotomy location is correct.

- Meticulous post-operative strapping is needed to ensure deformity correction is maintained during the healing period.

- Percutaneous hammer toe corrections have shown good short-term outcomes;[3,24] however, long-term studies with larger populations are required.[3]

DISCLOSURE

The authors have nothing to disclose.

REFERENCES

1. Ellington JK. Hammertoes and clawtoes: proximal interphalangeal joint correction. Foot Ankle Clin 2011;16(4):547–58.
2. Dunn JE, Link CL, Felson DT, et al. Prevalence of foot and ankle conditions in a multiethnic community sample of older adults. Am J Epidemiol 2004;159(5):491–8.
3. Mateen S, Raja S, Casciato DJ, et al. Minimally invasive versus open hammertoe correction: a retrospective comparative study. J Foot Ankle Surg 2023. https://doi.org/10.1053/j.jfas.2023.09.014. Published online October 6.
4. Coughlin MJ. Lesser toe abnormalities. Instr Course Lect 2003;52:421–44.
5. Malhotra K, Davda K, Singh D. The pathology and management of lesser toe deformities. EFORT Open Rev 2016;1(11):409–19.
6. Gregg J, Marks P, Silberstein M, et al. Histologic anatomy of the lesser metatarsophalangeal joint plantar plate. Surg Radiol Anat 2007;29(2):141–7.
7. Deland JT, Lee KT, Sobel M, et al. Anatomy of the plantar plate and its attachments in the lesser metatarsal phalangeal joint. Foot Ankle Int 1995;16(8):480–6.
8. Johnston RB, Smith J, Daniels T. The plantar plate of the lesser toes: an anatomical study in human cadavers. Foot Ankle Int 1994;15(5):276–82.
9. Jha S, Clark C. Plantar plate rupture: aetiology, diagnosis and treatment. Orthop Trauma 2023;37(1):28–33.
10. Maas NMG, van der Grinten M, Bramer WM, et al. Metatarsophalangeal joint stability: a systematic review on the plantar plate of the lesser toes. J Foot Ankle Res 2016;9:32.

11. Darcel V, Piclet-Legré B. Lesser-toe deformity. Orthop Traumatol Surg Res 2023; 109(1S):103464.
12. Schuberth JM. Hammer toe syndrome. J Foot Ankle Surg 1999;38(2):166–78.
13. Dhukaram V, Hossain S, Sampath J, et al. Correction of hammer toe with an extended release of the metatarsophalangeal joint. J Bone Joint Surg Br 2002; 84(7):986–90.
14. Coughlin MJ, Mann RA. Surgery of the foot and ankle. Incorporated: Mosby; 1999.
15. Coughlin MJ, Baumfeld DS, Nery C. Second MTP joint instability: grading of the deformity and description of surgical repair of capsular insufficiency. Phys Sportsmed 2011;39(3):132–41.
16. Feuerstein CA, Weil L Jr, Weil LS, et al. Static versus dynamic musculoskeletal ultrasound for detection of plantar plate pathology. Foot Ankle Spec 2014;7(4): 259–65.
17. Sung W, Weil L Jr, Weil LS, et al. Diagnosis of plantar plate injury by magnetic resonance imaging with reference to intraoperative findings. J Foot Ankle Surg 2012;51(5):570–4.
18. Albright RH, Brooks BM, Chingre M, et al. Diagnostic accuracy of magnetic resonance imaging (MRI) versus dynamic ultrasound for plantar plate injuries: a systematic review and meta-analysis. Eur J Radiol 2022;152:110315.
19. Federer AE, Tainter DM, Adams SB, et al. Conservative management of metatarsalgia and lesser toe deformities. Foot Ankle Clin 2018;23(1):9–20.
20. Formosa C, Grixti C, Gatt A. Conservative approach in the management of lesser toe deformities in older adults. J Am Podiatr Med Assoc 2022;112(3). https://doi.org/10.7547/20-274.
21. Albright RH, Hassan M, Randich J, et al. Risk factors for failure in hammertoe Surgery. Foot Ankle Int 2020;41(5):562–71.
22. De Prado M, Cuervas-Mons M, Golan'o P, Vaquero J. Distal metatarsal minimal invasive osteotomy (DMMO) for the treatment of metatarsalgia. Tech Foot Ankle Surg 2016;15(1):12–8.
23. Redfern DJ, Vernois J. Percutaneous Surgery for metatarsalgia and the lesser toes. Foot Ankle Clin 2016;21(3):527–50.
24. Yassin M, Garti A, Heller E, et al. Hammertoe correction with K-wire fixation compared with percutaneous correction. Foot Ankle Spec 2017;10(5):421–7.

Complex Forefoot Reconstruction with Percutaneous Techniques

Eric S. Baskin, DPM

KEYWORDS

- Minimally invasive foot surgery • Metatarsus adductus • DMMO
- Percutaneous metatarsal osteotomy • Hammer toes • Metatarsalgia

KEY POINTS

- Reconstruction of complex forefoot deformities using percutaneous MIS.
- MIS osteotomy orientation and technique.
- MIS anatomic long axis of the metatarsal (ALAM).
- MIS transverse and sagittal plane complex forefoot techniques.
- MIS reconstruction of metatarsus adductus with or without minimally invasive bunion surgery (MIBS).

INTRODUCTION

Complex forefoot deformities are some of the toughest challenges that a foot surgeon faces in the operating room. Surgical management is extremely labor intensive requiring extensive planning and technical proficiency to meet the demands of the pathology. Often the surgeon is greeted with distorted anatomy after making the incision, which has manifested over many years. Deformities over long periods of time cause cartilaginous structures, tendons, and ligaments to morph into unusual positions. To correct these deformities with an open approach requires a mammoth undertaking. However, with new minimally invasive surgery (MIS), the correction of these complex deformities is easier on the surgeon and the patient.

Advantages of MIS of the forefoot include the ability to correct complex deformities at the extracapsular and extraarticular levels. One can make a correction proximal and/or distal to the apex of deformity with minimal disruption to the joints and soft tissue structures. This preserves joint motion, produces less scarring, allows immediate weight bearing, and produces less pain postoperatively.

1322 Route 72, Suite 3, Manahawkin, NJ 08050, USA
E-mail address: drericbaskin@hotmail.com

Clin Podiatr Med Surg 42 (2025) 47–60
https://doi.org/10.1016/j.cpm.2024.05.001   **podiatric.theclinics.com**
0891-8422/25/© 2024 Elsevier Inc. All rights are reserved, including those for text and data mining, AI training, and similar technologies.

SOFT TISSUE BALANCING OF THE METATARSAL PHALANGEAL JOINT

Addressing soft tissue imbalances of the forefoot with a scalpel involves precise movements to address soft tissue contractures without disrupting normal soft tissue structures. It is recommended to use an instrument designed for tight spaces, such as #64 or #67 blade. In almost every complex metatarsal phalangeal joint (MPJ) contracture, percutaneous tenotomies of the extensor tendons and capsulotomies of the dorsal aspect of the MPJ are performed. Typically, this is done before carrying out the osseous work. This is accomplished through a stab incision 5 mm proximal to the MPJ and sliding the scalpel blade underneath and perpendicular to the extensor tendons. With the serrated edge pressing up against the plantar surface of the tendon, the toe is plantarflexed at the MPJ until the tenotomy is completed. The blade is then advanced subcutaneously distally toward the MPJ capsule and then inserted into the dorsal aspect of the joint. With a transverse sweeping motion, the capsulotomy is completed. The toe is once again plantarflexed to complete the correction. In the case of transverse plane deformities at the MPJ, the medial or lateral capsule is then released depending on the side of the contracture, and the noncontracted side is ultimately left intact. Continuing in stepwise fashion, the digital deformities distal to the MPJ are addressed with a combination of percutaneous tenotomies, capsulotomies, osteotomies, and/or digital joint arthrodesis. After completing the digital corrections, the surgeon determines if a metatarsal osteotomy is needed, and which type is most appropriate.

PRINCIPLES OF LESSER METATARSAL OSTEOTOMY ORIENTATION

Repairing complex deformities of the forefoot is categorized into procedures that address the transverse plane and sagittal plane pathology. The orientation of the metatarsal osteotomy is tailored to correct each plane of deformity.

Sagittal Plane

The orientation of the lesser metatarsal osteotomy (**Fig. 1**) in the sagittal plane is traditionally from dorsal distal to proximal plantar. It is recommended to use an instrument designed for these purposes, such as a 2 × 12 Shannon bur with low speed/high torque power console. The more acute the angle of the osteotomy, the more superior translation one can obtain of the head with less potential for shortening. An acutely angled osteotomy may be of benefit in neuropathic ulcers or with a plantarly displaced malunion of the metatarsal head. Conversely, the more obtuse the osteotomy in the sagittal plane, the more shortening and less potential for metatarsal elevation occurs. Obtuse osteotomies in the sagittal plane are helpful in cases of elongated metatarsals. Shortening in these circumstances may be necessary to address the pathologic transverse or sagittal plane malalignment of the metatarsal.

Transverse Plane

The orientation of the lesser metatarsal osteotomy (see **Fig. 1**) in the transverse plane is driven by the position of the tip of the bur in relationship to the anatomic long axis of the metatarsal (ALAM). If the tip of the bur is perpendicular to the ALAM in the transverse plane, then the osteotomy theoretically will be neutral and have less of a tendency to move in the transverse plane. If the tip of the bur is orientated oblique to the ALAM, then the osteotomy will proceed in that direction. This can influence the transverse plane correction and the amount of shortening that takes place at the metatarsal. Therefore, the more oblique the osteotomy is performed in the transverse plane,

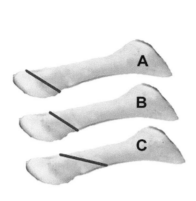 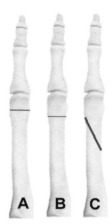

Fig. 1. Osteotomy configurations of the various MIS lesser metatarsal osteotomies. (*A*) Distal intracapsular metatarsal osteotomy. (*B*) Distal metaphyseal metatarsal osteotomy. (*C*) Distal oblique metaphyseal metatarsal osteotomy.

the greater the potential for shortening and transverse plane correction available (**Fig. 2**).

MINIMALLY INVASIVE SURGERY LESSER METATARSAL OSTEOTOMIES

Malalignment of a metatarsal may occur secondary to retrograde forces at the MPJ from a malpositioned digit. Therefore, digital pathology is corrected before metatarsal pathology if present. The main goals of a lesser metatarsal osteotomy are to relieve plantar pain and improve the position and function of the digit. Although traditional attention is focused on the lengths of the metatarsals with two-dimensional standard radiographs, restoring the metatarsal parabola pressures of the forefoot frontal plane arch is necessary to prevent transfer metatarsalgia.[1,2] If possible, it is preferable to accomplish these goals without ever operating on the metatarsal itself. An example of this would be to stabilize medial column insufficiency via hallux valgus repair and/or perform hammertoe repairs to reduce overloading and retrograde forces at the MPJ, in lieu of performing lesser metatarsal osteotomies.[3] If appropriate, this option avoids the potential downsides of lesser metatarsal MIS, such as prolonged overall healing, edema, and overall related complication risks.

DISTAL METAPHYSEAL METATARSAL OSTEOTOMY

The distal metaphyseal metatarsal osteotomy (DMMO), first described by De Prado and colleagues in 2004, is an extra-articular lesser metatarsal neck osteotomy with an orientation of 45° degrees.[4–6] An inherent advantage to the procedure is the lack of fixation, which allows the metatarsal to "self-adjust" during weight bearing (**Figs. 3** and **4**).[7] The osteotomy configuration allows for simultaneous shortening and elevation. There is increased risk of nonunion and transfer metatarsalgia if the procedure is performed in isolation.[8] Therefore, multiple osteotomies are traditionally performed contiguously on pathologic and nonpathologic metatarsals 2, 3, and 4 to balance the ground reactive forces through the distal forefoot. Shortening of the DMMO is approximately 4 mm.

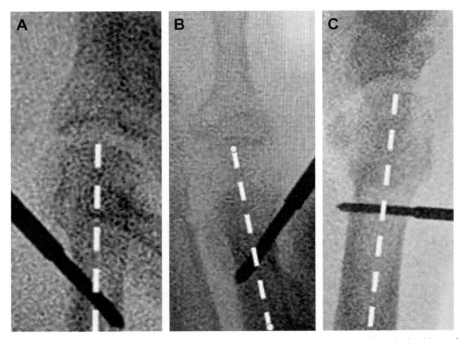

Fig. 2. Schematic of the anatomic long axis of the metatarsal (ALAM) in *white dashed line*. If the tip of the bur is oblique to the ALAM, then the osteotomy will follow that path in the transverse plane. The more oblique the osteotomy is, the more the head will move transversely and shorten (*A, B*). If the tip of the bur is perpendicular to the ALAM, then the osteotomy will be neutral and will have less of a tendency to move in the transverse plane and shorten (*C*).

In the presence of hallux valgus and medial column insufficiency, performing DMMOs may lead to recurrence of both pathologies (**Fig. 5**). The inherent orientation of the flexor and extensor digitorum tendons tend to translate the lesser metatarsal heads 2 to 4 laterally. This may not occur intraoperatively, but does occur in the postoperative period during weight bearing. Sometimes this lateral translation of the head is excessive causing an iatrogenic increase in the 1st and 2nd intermetatarsal angle. This phenomenon can lead to the start of hallux valgus (**Fig. 6**), exacerbation of an existing hallux valgus deformity, or recurrence of a recent surgically corrected hallux valgus deformity.[9] It is the author's opinion that excessive postoperative weight bearing, peripheral neuropathy, and improper bandaging increase the recurrence risk. In addition, a sagittal plane DMMO malunion can occur causing metatarsalgia and recurrence, which is more common in cavus feet because of the plantarly declinated metatarsals. Transverse malunion can cause undesirable angulation of the lesser digits at the MPJ. Sagittal plane malunion may result in loss of digital purchase and in situations where this might be a postoperative risk, the surgeon should consider more proximal metatarsal osteotomy.

DISTAL INTRACAPSULAR METATARSAL OSTEOTOMY

The distal intracapsular metatarsal osteotomy, an intracapsular osteotomy, has the benefit of less shortening and transverse plane movement because of a restraining

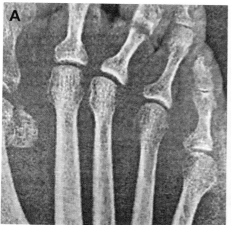 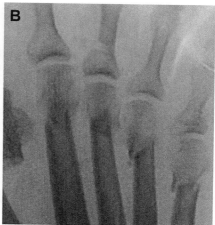

Fig. 3. Example of MIS lesser metatarsal osteotomies. (*A*) Preoperative anteroposterior radiograph demonstrating different osteotomy orientations needed to adjust for metatarsal length and restoration of the abnormal parabola. (*B*) Fluoroscopic image illustrating a normal metatarsal parabola after various lesser metatarsal osteotomies. The 2nd metatarsal osteotomy is an example of a DMMO made perpendicular to the ALAM, so minimal translatory transverse plane movement or shortening will occur. The 3rd and 4th DOMMOs were performed obliquely to the ALAM, which facilitates translatory transverse plane movement and shortening. The orientation of the 3rd DOMMO was oriented to translate proximal and lateral. The orientation of the 4th DOMMO was oriented to translate in the proximal and medial direction. The 5th metatarsal translates medially despite having the osteotomy performed perpendicular to ALAM. This is caused by the inherent medial pull and orientation of the long flexor and extensor tendons on the 5th toe.

effect of the capsule. Because the metatarsal head is less likely to overdrift, it is the author's opinion that it is best suited when an isolated shortening and elevation second metatarsal osteotomy needs to be performed in the presence of hallux valgus (**Fig. 7**). When compared with other MIS lesser metatarsal osteotomies, the distal intracapsular metatarsal osteotomy may have increased risks of nonunion/delayed union, iatrogenic arthritis, stiffness of the MPJ, and inadequate correction. The osteotomy can relieve plantar pressures under the metatarsal because of the mild shortening and mild elevation of the head.

DISTAL OBLIQUE METAPHYSEAL METATARSAL OSTEOTOMY

The distal oblique metaphyseal metatarsal osteotomy (DOMMO) was originally described in Bucharest, Romania by Marius Uscatu (unpublished data). It is performed obliquely in sagittal and transverse planes. The actual location of this osteotomy is at the metaphyseal and/or diaphyseal region of the lesser metatarsals. The main differences between the DOMMO and the DMMO include the increased amount of metatarsal shortening that DOMMO yields (up to 1 cm in some instances).[10] The DOMMO also affords much greater control of the osteotomy in the transverse plane. Performing a longer osteotomy lends to more shortening with greater bone-to-bone contact.

The DOMMO is advantageous in cases of metatarsus adductus (MA), grossly elongated lesser metatarsals with digital deformities, and with complex severe

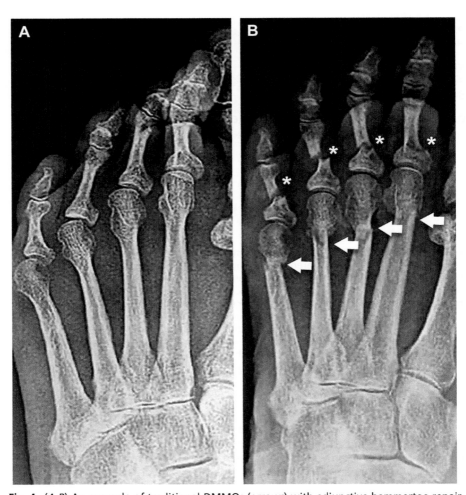

Fig. 4. (*A,B*) An example of traditional DMMOs (*arrows*) with adjunctive hammertoe repair via proximal phalangeal osteotomies (*asterisks*). Lateral drift and shortening of the 2nd and 3rd metatarsals occur because of the inherent lateral orientation of the long flexor and extensor tendons on the respective toes. In this particular case, the 4th metatarsal head translated medially based on the retrograde forces placed on it by the associated repair of the 4th digit. As previously stated, isolated medial translation of the 5th metatarsal head occurs almost all the time.

transverse plane deformities (**Fig. 8**). When hallux valgus exists with severe MA, the DOMMO and it's more proximal osteotomy allows lateral translation of the lesser metatarsals with a concomitant minimally invasive bunion surgery (MIBS), by removing the inherent lesser metatarsal blocking of the first metatarsal correction (**Figs. 9** and **10**). The distal location of the traditional DMMO blocks the first metatarsal head lateral translation, and therefore is not of benefit in hallux valgus correction in the face of MA with a low intermetatarsal angle. The downside to the DOMMO technique is prolonged edema, delayed overall healing, increased nonunion risk, malunion, undercorrection, and potential for excessive elevation.

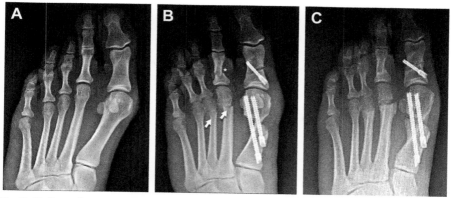

Fig. 5. Hallux valgus recurrence can occur after simultaneous MIBS and MIS MA correction when the location of the lesser metatarsal osteotomy is not proximal enough. This in turn blocks the lateralization of the first metatarsal head. (*A*) Preoperative anteroposterior radiograph with a large hallux valgus deformity and associated symptomatic MA. (*B*) Post-operative 2-week radiographs after MIBS, DMMO 2nd and 3rd metatarsals (*arrows*), and second toe realignment via proximal phalanx osteotomy (*asterisk*). The bunion correction seems to be adequate at this juncture in time. (*C*) Final healed radiographs demonstrate minor recurrence of the hallux valgus, likely because of not performing the lesser metatarsal osteotomies proximally enough. Instead of being able to move the forefoot as a unit, the first metatarsal head had some of its correction blocked by the second metatarsal shaft.

As an alternative, one can opt to perform closing wedge osteotomies at the proximal metaphyseal portion of the metatarsals.[11] Although this osteotomy has all the benefits of the DOMMO in the transverse plane, it does not have the shortening capacity that the DOMMO is known for.

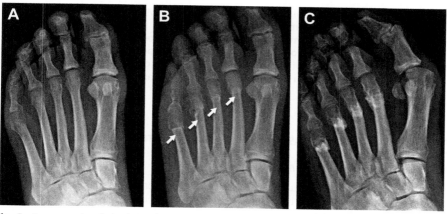

Fig. 6. An example of the lateralization of DMMOs leading to iatrogenic hallux valgus. (*A*) Preoperative radiograph. (*B*) Postoperative radiograph after lesser metatarsal DMMOs (*arrows*) for the treatment of metatarsalgia. (*C*) Healed radiograph with shortened and laterally translated metatarsals after DMMOs have led to the development of a hallux valgus deformity with an increased intermetatarsal angle.

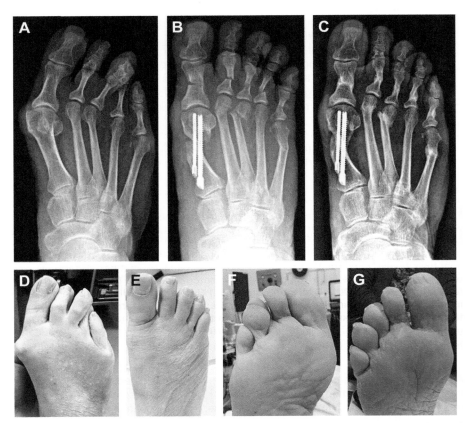

Fig. 7. An example of a distal intracapsular metatarsal osteotomy performed on the 2nd metatarsal to prevent lateralization during hallux valgus repair. (*A*) Preoperative radiograph. (*B*) Two weeks postoperative: DOMMO is performed on the 3rd metatarsal with the bur tip aimed lateral and proximal to the ALAM to enhance shortening and lateralization of the osteotomy. Adjunctive hammertoe procedures were performed before the metatarsal osteotomies. (*C*) Eight months postoperative. (*D*) Preoperative dorsal clinical presentation. (*E*) Postoperative dorsal clinical presentation. (*F*) Preoperative plantar clinical presentation with plantar callosity. (*G*) Postoperative plantar clinical presentation. Note the correction of the 4th digit clinically and resolution of the plantar callosity.

ADVANCED MINIMALLY INVASIVE SURGERY FOREFOOT TECHNIQUES IN COMPLEX CLINICAL SCENARIOS
Malunion Revision of Lesser Metatarsals

Whether it is iatrogenic or traumatically induced, the repair of lesser metatarsal malunions is treated with MIS. Using the osteotomy principles previously mentioned, the surgeon may orient the bur tip in the sagittal and/or transverse plane to dial in the correction. A common example is when correcting a plantar lateral metatarsal malunion. One can perform a DMMO with an acute angle in the sagittal plane and the bur tip obliquely medial to the ALAM. This acts to facilitate dorsiflexion and medialization of the metatarsal head.

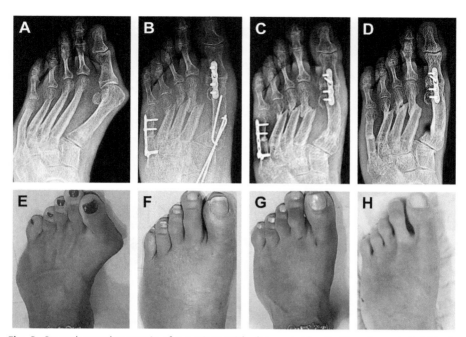

Fig. 8. Staged complex repair of a patient with rheumatoid arthritis using a hybrid technique of open and MIS. The first stage required traditional open hindfoot varus and peroneal tendon surgery. Stage 2 required an MPJ fusion with a mini-open proximal chevron bunionectomy. (*A*) Preoperative radiograph. (*B*) Two-week postoperative radiograph: The provisional fixation in the 1st metatarsal proximal chevron osteotomy had to be backed out after it was observed intraoperatively that the 2nd metatarsal was blocking the lateral translation and correction of the 1st metatarsal head. DOMMO was performed on metatarsals 2 to 5. The 5th metatarsal needed to be opened up and fixated. The definitive correction and fixation of the proximal chevron osteotomy and first MPJ fusion were performed after the lesser metatarsal work had been completed. (*C*) Six-month postoperative radiograph. The 5th metatarsal plate was removed 12 months postoperative. (*D*) Fourteen-month postoperative radiograph. (*E*) Preoperative clinical presentation. (*F*) Two-week postoperative clinical presentation. (*G*) Six-month postoperative clinical presentation. (*H*) Fourteenmonth postoperative clinical presentation.

Recalcitrant Dorsal Metatarsal Phalangeal Joint Contracture

There are circumstances that require additional surgery to stabilize the MPJ beyond the scope of traditional digital surgery. Reducing the sagittal plane contracture at the MPJ may require advanced surgical procedures and decision making based on intraoperative findings.

Minimally invasive surgery only

Many times the sagittal plane contracture persists at the MPJ despite performing a proper soft tissue stepwise release and an adjunctive osseous digital repair. The joint may also be contracted in the transverse plane. At this point the surgeon may opt to hold off on performing an osteotomy and attempt to reduce the MPJ contracture while retrograding a 0.062 K-wire from the tip of the toe into the metatarsal head.[12] Once the joint is reduced the surgeon can now perform the appropriate lesser metatarsal osteotomy and the K-wire may be left in the metatarsal head for 4 to 6 weeks. It is

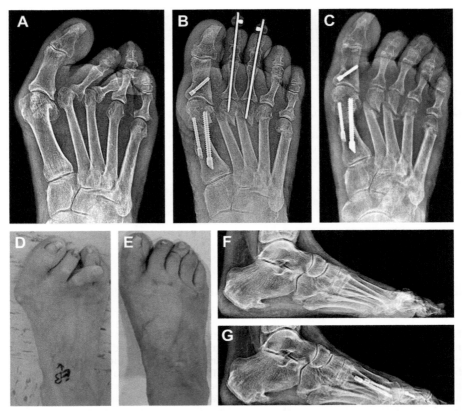

Fig. 9. An example of stabilizing the MPJ after percutaneous tendon balancing was performed with K-wires, before performing DOMMOs. (*A*) Preoperative anteroposterior (AP) radiograph. (*B*) Two-week postoperative AP radiograph. DOMMO of the 2nd and 3rd metatarsals were oriented lateral and proximal to the ALAM. Also noted is a DMMO with the orientation of the osteotomy performed perpendicular to the 4th metatarsal ALAM to prevent lateral drifting. (*C*) Ten-month AP postoperative radiograph. (*D*) Preoperative clinical presentation. (*E*) Ten-month postoperative clinical presentation. (*F*) Preoperative lateral radiograph. (*G*) Ten-month postoperative lateral radiograph.

important to make sure the K-wire does not interfere with the bur when performing the metatarsal osteotomy.

Mini-open

There are times when the MPJ does not reduce and/or is in a malposition after an attempt has been made to stabilize the joint with a retrograded 0.062 K-wire. When this occurs an open exploration is warranted and the surgeon must retract the K-wire to gain access for direct visualization of the MPJ. Traditional reduction and soft tissue release of the joint is performed and the surgeon may proceed by reinserting the K-wire into the metatarsal head, followed by performing the intended MIS metatarsal osteotomy.

Joint destruction

In rare instances when performing an open exploration of the MPJ the surgeon discovers that the anatomy of the joint is severely distorted by long-term gross cartilaginous adaptation and fibrosis. This advanced pathology prevents the proper reduction of the joint

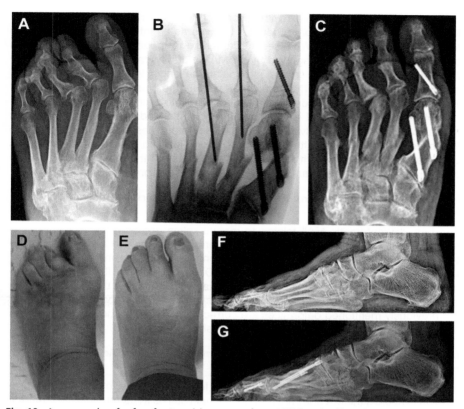

Fig. 10. An example of a forefoot revision case where MIBS and adjunctive DOMMOs were performed on metatarsals 2 to 4. (*A*) Preoperative AP radiograph. (*B*) Intraoperative AP radiograph. The osteotomies are placed proximal on the lesser metatarsals to prevent blocking of the 1st metatarsal head during translation. This technique may be used during the simultaneous correction of hallux valgus with severe irreducible metatarsus adductus. One must take into account the metatarsus adductus angle when addressing hallux valgus with metatarsus adductus to prevent undercorrection and recurrence. (*C*) Nineteen-month postoperative radiograph. (*D*) Preoperative clinical presentation. (*E*) Nineteen-month postoperative clinical presentation. (*F*) Preoperative lateral radiograph. (*G*) Nineteen-month postoperative lateral radiograph.

with the stepwise approach detailed previously. Alternatively, the surgeon may decide that the patient is better off with a joint destructive procedure, such as a 2-mm partial metatarsal head resection or a proximal phalanx base resection, performed with a sagittal saw, after which the newly reduced MPJ is promptly stabilized with the existing K-wire. At this point, the surgeon may proceed with a metatarsal osteotomy if warranted.

METATARSUS ADDUCTUS

Minimally invasive methods can treat MA through osteotomy rather than fusion. However, the mere presence of MA does not necessitate surgical correction.[13–16] It is common to observe MA resolution intraoperatively after digital deformity correction and elimination of the retrograde contracture forces. Therefore, one should correct the digital contracture deformities first before any lesser metatarsal osteotomy.

When evaluating hallux valgus with associated MA, it is important to consider the MA angle when preparing for surgery.[17] It serves as an intraoperative visual guide to prevent undercorrection. What seems like a mild-to-moderate bunion deformity is actually a large deformity disguised by an MA deformity on radiograph. It can give the optical illusion of a much smaller intermetatarsal angle. When MA has pathologic significance, correction is performed with or without the presence of hallux valgus.[18] There are several considerations that must be taken into account. The first is to determine if the MA is congenital or if it has developed secondary to retrograde forces placed on the MPJ from advanced hammertoe deformities. If it is congenital, the MA is less likely to reduce after hammertoe correction and/or bunion operation has been performed. In general, it is the author's opinion that the most practical way to determine this is to perform an intraoperative stepwise approach.

Intraoperative Stepwise Approach for Symptomatic Metatarsus Adductus without Hallux Valgus

The term "symptomatic MA" relates to metatarsalgia and advanced digital deformities. The initial step is to perform the hammertoe repairs to see if the digits reduce to a rectus position. In this case rectus is referring to the sagittal and transverse position of the toes clinically and fluoroscopically. One must also see if any plantar declination of the lesser metatarsal heads (metatarsalgia) persist after the toes have been corrected. Finally, the metatarsal parabola is inspected for pathology. If it is clear that the previously mentioned deformities are corrected and the parabola is normal, then addressing any residual MA with osteotomies should be avoided.

Intraoperative Stepwise Approach for Symptomatic Metatarsus Adductus with Hallux Valgus

If a hallux valgus deformity is present, then the first step is to perform MIBS with provisional fixation. If the MA does not reduce, the next step is to perform MIS hammertoe repairs as mentioned previously. If adequate translation of the first metatarsal osteotomy for hallux valgus correction is possible, and rectus position of the hammertoe repair is observed as mentioned previously, then addressing the MA is not necessary. If the appropriate amount of first metatarsal head lateral translation during MIBS cannot be completed, because of a blocking effect by the second metatarsal in adductus, and/or an inability to achieve a rectus position of the toes after hammertoe repairs are performed, then the MA should be considered for surgical resolution. At this point, the surgeon must back-out the MIBS provisional fixation and address the second metatarsal with a proximal metatarsal osteotomy, such as a DOMMO followed by osteotomies of the 3rd and 4th metatarsals of the surgeon's preference. This is necessary to complete the remainder of the operation. As detailed previously, after the DOMMO is performed one must take the MA angle into account, and the first metatarsal head is translated much further laterally than usual during MIBS to adjust for the MA angle and prevent undercorrection and recurrence.

BANDAGING AND POSTOPERATIVE COURSE

Although there is no set protocol, the principles of bandaging strive to stabilize the osteotomies and digital correction during weight bearing and the healing process. Adhesive strips are used to maintain digital correction while lengthwise folded gauze pads are placed in the interspaces and angled medially to stabilize hallux valgus repair if present, and prevent the metatarsal osteotomies from translating laterally. This technique is not written in stone and the surgeon should tailor the orientation of the interspace gauze dressings and digital taping to achieve the goals of the osteotomy. An example of this would be after the correction of MA, one may want to bandage the interspaces in a lateral orientation to maintain the lateral correction obtained from the osteotomies. The interdigital bandaging is then followed with a bulky dressing with light compression and surgical shoe. Dressing changes are suggested every 1 to 2 weeks until 6 weeks. At the 6 weeks, the patient can get the foot wet, return to a sneaker, and is taught to tape the digits on their own for an additional 4 more weeks. Physical therapy is used on an as-needed basis at the discretion of the surgeon.

SUMMARY

Percutaneous lesser metatarsal osteotomies are a powerful tool used to correct complex forefoot deformities. There are clear benefits of an MIS approach (over large incisional approaches) because of the limited disruption of the soft tissues, ability to bear weight immediately, less pain, and a quicker rehabilitation process. The real gift of MIS to us as surgeons is the ability to channel and use the ground reactive forces during weight bearing to our advantage. This allows us to tailor our osteotomy correction to each patient's anatomy and unique gait. However, not every complex case can be managed entirely with MIS. This genre of surgery requires proper didactic education, cadaver laboratory participation, and above all, a fair amount of MIS experience. It is imperative when addressing complex deformities that the surgeon considers using a combination of open and percutaneous techniques (hybrid) to achieve the optimal surgical result. A common mistake surgeons can make early in their minimally invasive learning journey is to commit entirely to a percutaneous approach, only to revisit the operating room a year later to redo or a touch-up a surgery that could have been previously addressed with an open surgical procedure.

CLINICS CARE POINTS

- Proper MIS didactic education, cadaveric training, and experience are essential prerequisites before performing these advanced techniques on a patient.
- Position of the bur to the ALAM drives the orientation of the osteotomy.
- MIS osteotomies tend to drift laterally without fixation. This can cause iatrogenic hallux valgus or diminish the result of an existing bunionectomy. The orientation of the osteotomy can lessen or prevent this phenomenon.
- Surgical management of metatarsus adductus is not always necessary and should be approached in a stepwise fashion intraoperatively.
- When performing MIBS together with MIS correction of MA one must take the metatarsus adductus angle into account.
- MIS combined with traditional open techniques (hybrid) is sometimes necessary to achieve the optimal result.

DISCLOSURE

The author has nothing to disclose.

REFERENCES

1. Barouk P. Recurrent metatarsalgia. Foot Ankle Clin 2014;19:407–24.

2. Feibel JB, Tisdel CL, Donley BD. Lesser metatarsal osteotomies. A biomechanical approach to metatarsalgia. Foot Ankle Clin 2001;6:473–89.
3. Lee KB, Park JK, Park YH, et al. Prognosis of painful plantar callosity after hallux valgus correction without lesser metatarsal osteotomy. Foot Ankle Int 2009;30: 1048–52.
4. De Prado M, Ripoll PL, Golano P. Cirurgìa percutanea del pie. The Netherlands: Elsevier España, S.L.U.; 2004.
5. Coillard JY, Laffenetre O, Cermolacce C. et. al. Percutaneous treatment of static metatarsalgia with distal metatarsal mini-invasive osteotomy. In: Maffulli N, Easley M, editors. Minimally Invasive Surgery of the Foot and Ankle. New York, NY: Springer; 2011. p. 163–9.
6. Coillard J.Y., DMMO. Cazeau C. Chirurgie mini-invasive et percutanée du pied, vol 2. Sauramps medical, Montpellier, DL, 2015, cop. 2015. 219-240.
7. Laffenêtre O, Perera A. Distal minimally invasive metatarsal osteotomy ("DMMO"-Procedure). Foot Ankle Clin 2019;24:615–25.
8. Johansen JK, Jordan M, Thomas M. Clinical and radiological outcomes after Weil osteotomy compared to distal metatarsal metaphyseal osteotomy in the treatment of metatarsalgia: a prospective study. Foot Ankle Surg 2019;25:488–94.
9. Henry J, Besse JL, Fessy MH. Distal osteotomy of the lateral metatarsals: a series of 72 cases comparing the Weil osteotomy and the DMMO percutaneous osteotomy. Orthop Traumatol Surg Res 2011;97:S57–65.
10. Laffenêtre Olivier. France, Personal conversation 2018.
11. Burg A, Palmanovich E. Correction of severe hallux valgus with metatarsus adductus applying the concepts of minimally invasive surgery. Foot Ankle Clin 2020;25(2):337–43.
12. Piclet-Legré B. Lesser-toe deformities. Orthop Traumatol Surg Res 2021. https://doi.org/10.1016/j.otsr.2022.103464. MIS Global Conference for Foot Surgery.
13. Dawoodi AI, Perera A. Reliability of metatarsus adductus angle and correlation with hallux valgus. Foot Ankle Surg 2012;18(3):180–6.
14. Kurashige T. Minimally invasive surgery for severe hallux valgus with severe metatarsus adductus: foot Ankle Surg. Techn, Rep Cases 2021;1(1):100007.
15. Chomej P, Klos K, Bauer S, et al. Lateralising DMMO (MIS) for simultaneous correction of a pes adductus during surgical treatment of a hallux valgus. Foot 2020;45(1).
16. Aiyer A, Shub J, Shariff R, et al. Radiographic recurrence of deformity after hallux valgus surgery in patients with metatarsus adductus. Foot Ankle Int 2016;37(2): 165–71.
17. Loh B, Chen JY, Yew AKS. Prevalence of metatarsus adductus in symptomatic hallux valgus and its influence on functional outcome. Foot Ankle Int 2015;36(11): 1316–21.
18. Aiyer AA, Shariff R, Ying L, et al. Prevalence of metatarsus adductus in patients undergoing hallux valgus surgery. Foot Ankle Int 2014;35(12):1292–7.

Percutaneous Lapidus Bunionectomy

A New, Less Invasive Method for a 100 Year Old Surgery

Joel Vernois, MD[a,b,*], David Redfern, MD[c,d], Eric S. Baskin, DPM[e]

KEYWORDS

- Lapidus • Percutaneous • Mini-invasive surgery • Hallux valgus • Flat feet

KEY POINTS

- Lapidus can be done percutaneously.
- It is an effective procedure to correct all severities of hallux valgus.
- The procedure requires specific comprehensive training in percutaneous techniques.
- Industry-manufactured jigs may assist the surgeon through the learning curve.
- Resection of all of the cartilage on both sides of the joint is essential to mitigating nonunion.

INTRODUCTION

Hallux abductovalgus deformity of the first ray is common with a large variety of options for surgical treatment utilizing open surgical techniques. Since described by Albrecht and Lapidus almost 100 years ago, first tarsometatarsal joint (TMTJ) fusion has become a common procedure in the treatment of bunion deformity.[1,2] Named after the author, the Lapidus (procedure) is an effective technique that can control the position of the first metatarsal in 3 different planes.[3–6] Since its inception in the 1930s, there have been many modifications and variations to the original Lapidus procedure. Recently, the popularity of the Lapidus procedure has dramatically increased as a surgical option for hallux valgus. Contemporary belief is of the opinion that the apex of the hallux abductovalgus deformity originates at the first TMTJ.[7–11] The Lapidus procedure allows the surgeon to address severe deformities, while providing a

[a] ICP, Clinique Blomet, 136bis rue Blomet, Paris 75015, France; [b] Sussex Orthopaedic NHS Treatment Centre, Lewes Road, Haywards Heath, England; [c] Cleveland Clinic London, 33 Grosvenor Place, London SW1x 7HY; [d] Montefiore Hospital, Hove, East Sussex, England; [e] Advocare Stafford Orthopedics, Manahawkin, NJ 08050, USA
* Corresponding author.
E-mail address: Joel.vernois@sfr.fr

Clin Podiatr Med Surg 42 (2025) 61–75
https://doi.org/10.1016/j.cpm.2024.08.001
0891-8422/25/© 2024 Elsevier Inc. All rights reserved, including those for text and data mining, AI training, and similar technologies.
podiatric.theclinics.com

stable and reliable fixation construct during healing.[12] First TMTJ fusion has been reported to lower the risk of recurrence, particularly in patients with first TMTJ joint hypermobility.[13] Arthrodesis of the first TMTJ can also be used for the surgical management of various deformities of the foot including hallux limitus, hypermobility of the first TMTJ, arthritis of the first TMTJ, and as an integral part of flatfoot reconstruction.

Inherent risks are ever present in traditional open Lapidus surgery including wound healing complications, nonunion, malunion, delayed healing, and painful hardware removal.[14–16] The first TMTJ has a curvature and is one of the deepest joints in the foot which makes it difficult to perform an open arthrodesis. Surgeons can risk removing too much bone during joint resection resulting in first-ray shortening, which can be worse when the surgeon performs plantar cuts to accommodate for extreme angular deformities. Average first metatarsal shortening has been reported to be from 2.9 mm to as high as 8.0 mm with open techniques and 2.7 mm with minimally invasive (MI) techniques.[17,18] Nonunion is one of the most frequent major complications that can occur after open first TMTJ fusion, and its incidence has been reported from 2% to 10%.[19,20] In an effort to improve outcomes and decrease complication rates, MI techniques have been implemented for the Lapidus procedure.[21,22]

With the recent resurgence of new minimally invasive bunion surgery (MIBS) involving distal metatarsal osteotomy procedures, there has been a revival of minimally invasive surgery (MIS) in the foot as a whole, and the Lapidus procedure is no exception. The well-known benefits of MI techniques involve minimal soft tissue disruption and immediate weight bearing after select procedures[23–25] (**Box 1**). As such, percutaneous Lapidus techniques being described in the literature and performed in more regularity by the MI surgical community (**Figs. 1** and **2**).

MI surgery and MIBS are not without their risks, which may include paraesthesia, tendon damage, nonunion, and malunion.[26,27] Furthermore, there is a well-known steep learning curve that poses a significant barrier to entry for many surgeons interested in MI procedures. Arthroscopic assisted surgery with that allows for direct visualization and percutaneous MIBS techniques using associated fluoroscopy have been reported.[28–31] Lui and colleagues[22] described this arthroscopic fusion of the first TMTJ performed through dorsal medial and plantar medial portals while using burs for the joint preparation. They experienced technical challenges resulting dorsiflexion, shortening, and first metatarsal adduction. Increased accuracy of the joint preparation would diminish these complications. The technique allowed the subchondral bone to remain intact, while avoiding excessive bone removal during the cartilaginous joint surface denuding process. The arthroscopic/percutaneous approach may minimize soft tissue damage, reduces postoperative pain, avoids restrictions on the osseous

---

Box 1
Benefits of percutaneous surgery

Less periosteal stripping.

Less pain.

Less soft tissue disruption.

Less instability due to the largely intact soft tissue envelope.

Early weight bearing postoperatively.

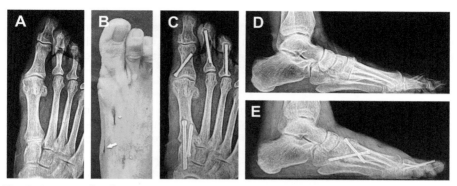

Fig. 1. An example of percutaneous Lapidus with Akin. (*A*) Preoperative anteroposterior radiograph and (*B*) intraoperative picture demonstrating percutaneous incisions. The portal for the bur is medial at the joint line (*white arrow*). The percutaneous fixation incisions (*asterisks*) are dorsally placed. (*C*) Postoperative anteroposterior radiograph demonstrating healed fusion site with 2 crossed screws. (*D*) Preoperative lateral radiograph and (*E*) postoperative anteroposterior lateral radiograph. (*Image Courtesy* of Kris Di Nucci, DPM.)

blood supply, decreases wound healing complications, and yields a better cosmetic result due to the small portals (**Fig. 3**).

In 2020, the senior authors of this study described a percutaneous technique for Lapidus arthrodesis using a bur and percutaneous chamfered screw fixation concluding that the technique is powerful, but excessive first ray shortening remains a major concern. MI approaches under direct fluoroscopic guidance have described a single portal technique on the medial aspect of the joint. Bean and colleagues[32] described early outcomes of percutaneous modified Lapidus with axial intramedullary nail technique compared to traditional open Lapidus. They found that the MI intramedullary group had a high union rate, lack of hardware failure, and tolerance for early weight bearing at 12 days post-surgery. The open group had higher complications rates, but the MI cohort showed a significantly higher rate of repeat surgery, which was attributed to the MI learning curve. They concluded that the technique may allow

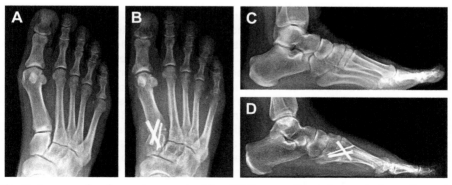

Fig. 2. An example of percutaneous Lapidus. (*A*) Preoperative anteroposterior radiograph demonstrating a mild/moderate bunion deformity. (*B*) Postoperative anteroposterior radiograph with fixation in place and rectus hallux. (*C*) Preoperative lateral radiograph and (*D*) postoperative lateral radiograph. (*Image Courtesy* of Jeffrey Dikis, DPM.)

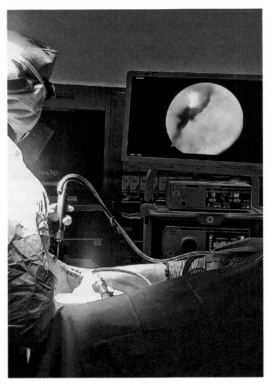

Fig. 3. Intraoperative picture during a combined arthroscopic/percutaneous first TMTJ arthrodesis with bur-assisted joint preparation. Use of the arthroscopic allows for direct arthroscopic visualization of cartilaginous resection. (*From*: Baskin ES, Luong K, Aamir A, Solomon M. Identification of portals and evaluation of their safeness for MIS arthrodesis of the 1st tarsometatarsal joint. Foot Ankle Surg: Techn, Rep Cases. 2023;3(1). With permission from.)

for a low rate of wound complications, accelerated rehabilitation, and improved cosmesis compared to the open Lapidus technique.

Another important study by Vieira and colleagues evaluated early radiographic results and complications of MI arthroscopic TMTJ arthrodesis compared to its open counterpart procedure in patients with hallux valgus deformity. The MI technique was performed utilizing medial and superomedial portals. A percutaneous lateral release and medial eminence resection were performed in conjunction with joint preparation using several burrs. A dorsal compression device was used to maintain correction through manual maneuvering and reduction. Percutaneous fixation in this study consisted of a partially threaded cannulated 3.5 mm intermetatarsal screw placed between the first and second metatarsals and 2 to 3 percutaneous fully threaded 4.0 mm cannulated crossing screws to transfix the TMTJ. All patients were heel weight bearing for the initial 2 weeks, then full weight bearing for 4 weeks in a boot. The study concluded that both the open and the MI techniques resulted in good to excellent correction, but the open group showed significantly greater radiographic correction of the intermetatarsal angle and hallux valgus angles.[16]

SURGICAL TECHNIQUE FOR MINIMALLY INVASIVE LAPIDUS

MI arthrodesis of the first TMTJ has several key steps and is challenging. Of course, adequate preparation of the joint surfaces is an important component in any joint arthrodesis to allow for proper osseous ingrowth at the joint fusion site. The most difficult challenge with MI resection of the first TMTJ is navigating the shape/curvatures of the joint, which is why the open extensile approaches have dominated Lapidus corrections. The specialized and burs that were developed for distal osteotomy MIBS are of great use with MI Lapidus and procedure-specific Lapidus tools are likely on the horizon. The percutaneous techniques call for incisions less than 5 mm that requires the use of low-speed/high-torque burs. A sagittal saw would not be able to properly navigate resection through such a small incision.

Another crucial step is the joint reduction maneuver that can be performed with or without external device jig assistance. It is important to follow the tenets of Lapidus correction requiring adequate reduction in the transverse, sagittal, and frontal planes to ensure proper correction and prevention of recurrence. The fixation is the last step in the surgery. Plates, staples, nails, and/or or screws can be utilized for fixation. However, when using percutaneous techniques, only screws or nails can be realistically implanted. The other forms of fixation may be employed when performing open or "mini-open" (smaller incisions) surgery but lose some of the benefits of percutaneous surgery. A fusion of the adjacent inter-cuneiform joint may also be undertaken with traditional percutaneous screw fixation.

Operating Room Setup

Operating room setup is very important with MI surgery, and particularly with Lapidus to provide access for the delivery of instruments and obtain proper radiographic imaging. The patient is positioned supine with the foot overhanging the end of the table. The position of the C-arm depends on your dominant hand. As a right-handed surgeon, the C-arm will be on the right side and the surgeon would stay on the left side of the operated foot, with the detector under the operative foot of the patient. A large or a small C-arm can be used. The knee on the nonoperative leg can be flexed with lateral support to exclude the nonoperative foot from the working area. The end position is where the foot is hanging off the table with C-arm plate directly below the foot (**Fig. 4**).

Instrumentation

The percutaneous technique requires specialized instruments (**Box 2**) and a fluoroscopic unit, which serve as the surgeon's eyes during the procedure. To prepare the joint, Shannon/wedge-type burs are used for cartilage resection. Angled rasps are used to clean the joint and remove all the cartilaginous debris. Fixation may vary but 4.0 mm screws are recommended by the authors.

Anesthesia

Surgery is performed under general anesthesia or regional peripheral block. Use of a tourniquet is not routine, especially if operating under an ankle block as this may be uncomfortable and painful for the patient. An advantage of not using a tourniquet is the potential cooling effect of the blood while you are using the rotary bur. A single dose of antibiotic is administered at induction of anesthesia.

Anatomic Considerations

Knowledge of the local anatomy and at-risk structures is paramount to the prevention of iatrogenic injury (**Fig. 5** and **Box 3**). Nerves are at particular risk for injury with portal

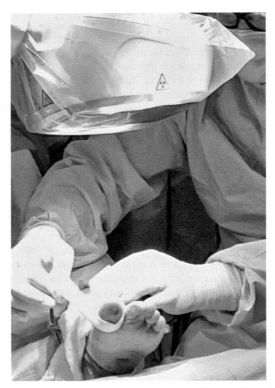

Fig. 4. Room setup involves the operative foot hanging off the edge of the table. The position of the C-arm is on the dominant hand side of the surgeon with the fluoroscopic detector plate under the foot.

placement and when the rotary bur flutes are in contact the nerve. The wedge bur is more aggressive and should be used judiciously when navigating important soft tissue structures.

Joint Preparation

Localization of the first TMTJ with the C-arm is the first step of this procedure. When preparing the joint, one must be very careful to avoid excessive bone resection.

Box 2
Specialized instruments for minimally invasive surgery

Beaver blade

Shannon bur of 20 mm length x 2 mm diameter

Shannon bur of 20 mm length x 3 mm diameter

Wedge bur of 12 mm length x 3 mm diameter

4.0 mm screws are recommended for fixation.

Fluoroscopic C-arm

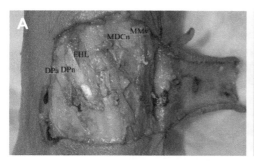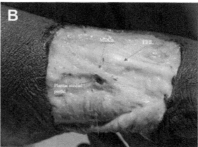

Fig. 5. Demonstration of the joint preparation of the 1st TMTJ without disruption of the anatomical structures. (*A*) Dissection around the dorsomedial and dorsolateral portal sites. (*B*) Dissection around plantar and medial portal sites. Note the structures that can be seen at risk; Extensor halluces longus tendon (EHL), medial dorsal cutaneous nerve (MDC).[33] (*From*: Baskin ES, Luong K, Aamir A, Solomon M. Identification of portals and evaluation of their safeness for MIS arthrodesis of the 1st tarsometatarsal joint. Foot Ankle Surg: Techn, Rep Cases. 2023;3(1). With permission from.)

Depending on the surgeon's preference and the rigidity of the joint, it may be necessary to utilize a biplanar lateral and plantarized wedge resection. In this situation, the authors recommend the use of 2 guiding K-wires to prevent excessive resection and wedge creation (**Figs. 6** and **7**). They will be placed from dorsal to plantar at the desired angle. The structures at risk lie on the dorsal side of the joint and lateral distal part of the joint.[33–35] Since the bur stays within the joint during the procedure, damage to the extra-articular structures should be at a minimum. Surgeons should mindfully stop use of the bur as soon as the dorsal or plantar capsule is reached. The position of the guiding K-wires must be carefully positioned to avoid damage to the superficial peroneal nerve or the dorsalis pedis artery. Placing the K-wires medial to the extensor tendon is preferable. When the joint is mobile and the deformity reducible, the use of K-wire guides may not be necessary.

The bur is introduced through a medial approach/portal placed over the middle of the joint, and the length of the incision should be kept below 10 mm. First, the Shannon bur (20 x 2 mm) is used as it is a slimmer bur and runs against each joint surface to resect the cartilage (**Fig. 8**). It is important to keep the bur within the joint and not deviate or wander extra-articularly. The rotation speed and the size of the portal are paramount to avoid any burning on the skin. A cooling system can be associated particularly if a tourniquet is inflated. The metatarsal-cuneiform capsular ligaments

---

Box 3
Important anatomic at-risk structures surrounding the first tarsometatarsal joint

Deep peroneal nerve

Dorsalis pedis artery

Tibialis anterior tendon

Extensor hallucis longus tendon

Adductor hallucis muscle

Medial dorsal cutaneous nerve

Medial marginal vein

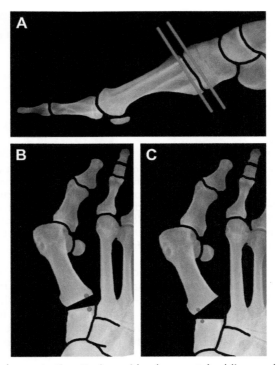

Fig. 6. Schematic demonstrating K-wire guide placement (*red lines* and *dots*). (*A*) Lateral view showing the periarticular placement of the K-wires to prevent excessive resection. (*B*) When the K-wires are laterally placed on the anteroposterior view, a modest wedge will be created. (*C*) When the K-wires are medially placed on the anteroposterior view, a larger wedge will be created.

must be released to allow the distraction of the TMTJ. The wedge burr is helpful to create perfect clean margins at the respective cartilage resection sites. It is necessary to take special care of the plantar region of the TMTJ, as some bone or cartilage can be easily left behind resulting in unwanted dorsiflexion malunion of the arthrodesis. Using the rasp, the debris should be regularly removed from the joint. When the joint is cleaned of cartilage, microfracture must be performed on both cuneiform and metatarsal bones, which can be performed with the Shannon bur (20 x 2 mm).

If the joint is rigid and immobile, a plantar and/or medial wedge might need to be performed, utilizing the K-wire guides as discussed earlier. The K-wire positions are very important and must be visualized carefully in both anteroposterior and lateral views. The plantar wedge is taken from the cuneiform bone rather than the metatarsal. For the lateral wedge, the position of the K-wires on the anteroposterior view is most critical. The more lateral the K-wire, the smaller the wedge (see **Fig. 4**A), the more medial the K-wire, the larger the wedge (see **Fig. 4**C). With this technique, the Shannon bur (20 x 3 mm) is used to follow the K-wires dorsally and plantarly. The authors prefer to start with the proximal K-wire. It is additional important to keep the bur perpendicular to the second metatarsal. When this first cut is complete, the joint becomes mobile and the intermetatarsal angle can then be corrected. The second cut along the distal K-wire is performed, but this cut is to be parallel to the first cut.

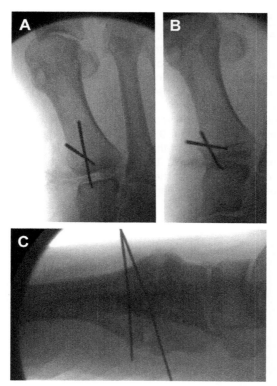

Fig. 7. Fluoroscopic series demonstrating guiding K-wire technique to prevent excessive resection of the TMTJ. Multiple radiographic views should be obtained to set the K-wires in the desired position. (*A*) Anteroposterior view, (*B*) oblique view, and (*C*) lateral view.

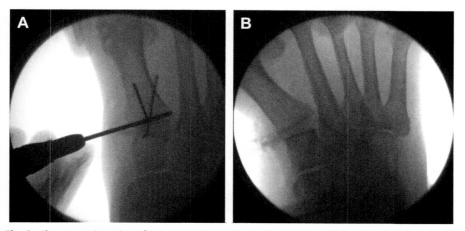

Fig. 8. Fluoroscopic series of joint resection using a Shannon bur (20 x 2 mm). (*A*) Note the bur remains in the confines of the guiding K-wires. (*B*) After joint resection.

Reduction Maneuver and Fixation

When the joint preparation is complete, the deformity is corrected utilizing the tenets of Lapidus surgery: reduction of the transverse, sagittal, and frontal planes. Once reduced, the joint is stabilized with provisional K-wires and/or cannulated screw guidewires. Fixation is traditionally performed by inserting a 4.0 mm cannulated screw obliquely from the distal dorsal first metatarsal to the proximal plantar aspect of the medial cuneiform. A second 4.0 mm cannulated screw is inserted from the dorsal proximal medial cuneiform and oriented distal and plantar to catch the plantar proximal part of the first metatarsal (**Fig. 9**). The authors recommend a distal horizontal screw positioned 3 to 4 cm distal to the joint line on the lateral side of the extensor tendon. The proximal screw would be inserted through a dorsal-lateral 5 mm approach to the extensor tendon. The stability of the fixation is assessed with a squeeze test (pressure with index finger and thumb between M1 and M2). If the

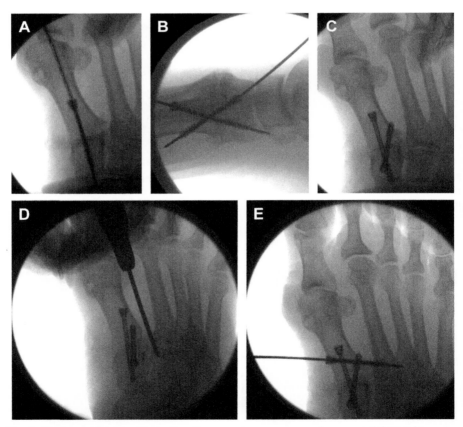

Fig. 9. Fluoroscopic series illustrating the percutaneous screw placement. (*A*) Distal to proximal screw is placed first. (*B*) Proximal to distal screw is placed using the lateral view. (*C*) The first TMTJ is secured with 2 compression screws. The squeeze test is performed to check for remaining intraoperative hypermobility—if present, then additional fusions may be indicated. (*D*) Percutaneous fusion between the first and second metatarsal bases demonstrated with a Shannon bur. (*E*) Percutaneous screw placement of a third screw for fusing the metatarsal bases together.

squeeze test shows an inter-cuneiform laxity, then a third screw is placed from medial to lateral between the first and the second metatarsal bases. The inter-cuneiform joint is then denuded with the wedge burr. A lateral release at the metatarsophalangeal joint is not systematic for the authors except if a retraction of the capsule is present. An Akin osteotomy is performed at the discretion of the surgeon.

Pitfalls with Guiding K-Wire Placement

The position and the orientation of the resectionary cuts are essential and rely on the position of the K-wires to achieve angular correction. If they are too medial, too much bone may be removed; too lateral then not enough bone is removed to obtain the correction. If one is not close enough to the joint, then too much bone may also be removed. Excessive shortening may result in lesser metatarsalgia even with the plantarflexory compensation at the head, which is why a short first metatarsal is probably not a good indication for a Lapidus. If the K-wires are parallel to each other, then the metatarsal cannot be plantarflexed. Divergent K-wires will allow the metatarsal head to be plantarflexed based on the amount of angulation between the 2 K-wires. The quality of the correction depends on the release of the TMTJ and the removal of the debris left in the joint particularly on the plantar part.

Jigs and Learning Curve

Different jigs are commercially available and may be helpful to assist the surgeon with the MI Lapidus technique. A distraction clamp can help to prepare the joint and remove all the debris while a reduction clamp assists in holding the joint in the desired reduction. This external provisional fixation frees up the surgeons hands to introduce the internal fixation. The authors recommend using the jig as an option at the beginning of the surgeon's learning curve to avoid excessive resection. It has also been shown during the learning curve that one can neglect the cartilage resection at the dorsal and lateral aspect of the TMTJ. Failure to completely resect the cartilage can result in nonunion and or malunion. In a cadaveric study by Baskin and colleagues[33], they concluded that direct arthroscopic visualization may improve outcomes by preventing inadequate joint preparation while facilitating proper removal of cartilaginous articular fragments within the joint.

POSTOPERATIVE MANAGEMENT

The postoperative care entails partial weight bearing in an orthopedic heel wedge shoe for 6 weeks with crutches. The dressing is removed 2 weeks after surgery. The patient follows up at 6 weeks and then 3 months. Return to sports including running is allowed after 3 months. Physiotherapy is at the discretion of the surgeon.

DISCUSSION

Lapidus has been used for nearly a century in the treatment of hallux valgus deformity with good and excellent results reported. The procedure is a versatile and powerful technique capable of correcting several deformities including hallux valgus.[8] Although popular, there are some difficult steps that must be recognized.

The preparation of the joint is central to the success of the procedure. With percutaneous technique, you cannot directly visualize the articular surfaces, and therefore, the surgeon cannot confirm the quality of the joint preparation (**Fig. 10**). They are fully reliant on assessing fluoroscopic views and clinical feel. The fluoroscopy can be misleading depending on the angle of the beam. It is also challenging to prepare a curved joint surface with a long and pointed straight bur. The authors recommend

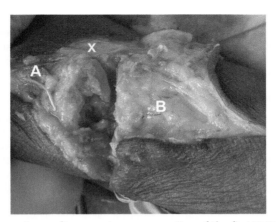

Fig. 10. Cadaveric specimen after percutaneous resection of the first TMTJ in a training lab. Inadequate cartilage resection can be seen here with much of the dorsal lateral cartilage remaining (X). (A) First metatarsal base. (B) Medial cuneiform. An incomplete resection of the cartilage from both sides of the joint may result in a nonunion or malunion.

alternating use of a straight bur with a smaller conical burr such as a 3.1 mm burr that is particularly useful for concave surfaces. Distraction of the joint with an external device can be helpful. If removing the cartilage seems easy, then one should be prepared to remove a minimum of the underlying sclerotic bone. This can be difficult in an arthritic joint and may lead to excessive resection. It is for this reason that the authors recommend the use of 2 K-wires to limit the amount of resection. Before fixing the 2 bones, microfractures are performed with the 20 mm x 2 mm burr on both the cuneiform and the metatarsal surfaces. Given the incidence of nonunion, it is vital that joint preparation is meticulous to minimize this risk.[36–38]

Some shortening of the first metatarsal is inevitable but can be minimized with experience and the use of the K-wires. Transfer metatarsalgia is another risk with this procedure. Lowering the metatarsal head (plantar wedge resection of cuneiform) should be considered in an effort to counteract the effects of metatarsal shortening while maintaining adequate first ray loading during gait. In essence, lowering the first metatarsal head is the solution to counteract shortening, but the final result also depends on other factors such as gastrocnemius tension/excursion and the patient's preferred footwear (eg, the daily use of heel shoe that will tend to overload the lesser metatarsals). The authors have not observed consequent metatarsalgia but remain mindful of this risk. This risk can also be related to the age of the patient and their activity. An index plus (longer metatarsal) would be less affected by the potential shortening. Conversely, an index minus (shorter metatarsal) is probably not a good indication for a Lapidus procedure. In this situation, a distal osteotomy would be the first choice. The alternative would be to associate a shortening osteotomy of the lateral metatarsals such as Weil osteotomies or distal metatarsal metaphyseal osteotomy (DMMO). Ideally, the DMMO requires immediate weight bearing that is not possible in the authors' postoperative regime. However, one may still perform DMMOs if there is sufficient intraoperative concern regarding the degree of shortening.

It is the author's opinion and preference that if a distal osteotomy MIBS is deemed possible/appropriate, then the Lapidus should be avoided. When a distal osteotomy is not deemed appropriate, a proximal procedure must be chosen. It is important to recognize that surgeons have different skill levels with MIBS and one surgeon might be able to correct severe bunion deformities in this manner where others might have to rely on Lapidus-fusion methods of angular bunion correction.

The fixation is an important part of Lapidus outcomes. Different implants can be used such as plates, screws, and/or nails. To date, percutaneous Lapidus-specific plates are not commercially available. Screws must be sited for optimal strength of fixation. If too dorsal, they offer the opportunity of a plantar gap during weight bearing. However, when placed plantar (as recommended earlier), they promote dorsal compression when weight bearing.

SUMMARY

The Lapidus is an important procedure for surgeons to have in their armamentarium. Now with the rise of MI surgery, the Lapidus procedure can now be performed in this manner. However, we are still at the infancy of the percutaneous Lapidus and the outcome studies are long off and the experience among surgeons is limited. The complications of shortening, nonunion, and malunion remain at the forefront regardless of MI versus open, and we recommend Lapidus-fusion bunionectomy be reserved for specific scenarios when a distal osteotomy MIBS is deemed unsuitable. In our opinion, learning and becoming proficient with percutaneous Lapidus technique are more challenging than other percutaneous techniques.

CLINICS CARE POINTS

- Use guiding K-wire technique to avoid excessive joint resection.
- Position and orientation of the joint resection/cut determine planar correction.
- Dorsal approach of the K-wire or the screws that can damaged the superficial peroneal nerve or the dorsal–medial artery.
- Excessive speed of the bur that can be burned the skin.

DISCLOSURE

The authors have nothing to disclose.

REFERENCES

1. Lapidus PW. A quarter of a century of experience with the operative correction of the metatarsus varus primus in hallux valgus. Bull Hosp Joint Dis 1956;17(2): 404–12.
2. Lapidus PW. The author's bunion operation from 1931 to 1959. Clin Orthop 1960; 16:119–35.
3. Dujela MD, Langan T, Cottom JM, et al. Lapidus arthrodesis. Clin Podiatr Med Surg 2022;39(2):187–220.
4. Lapidus PW. The operative correction of the metatarsus varus primus in hallux valgus. Surg Gynecol Obstet 1934;58:183, 191-7.
5. Li S, Myerson MS. Evolution of thinking of the lapidus procedure and fixation. Foot Ankle Clin 2020;25(1):109–12.
6. Vernois J, Redfern D, GRECMIP soon MIFAS. Lapidus, a percutaneous approach. Foot Ankle Clin 2020;25(3):407–12.
7. Baravarian B, Ben-Ad R. Contemporary approaches and advancements to the Lapidus procedure. Clin Podiatr Med Surg 2014;31(2):299–308.

8. Blitz NM. The versatility of the Lapidus arthrodesis. Clin Podiatr Med Surg 2009; 26(3):427–41.

9. King DM, Toolan BC. Associated deformities and hypermobility in hallux valgus: an investigation with weightbearing radiographs. Foot Ankle Int 2004;25:251–5.

10. Santrock RD, Smith B. Hallux valgus deformity and treatment: a three-dimensional approach: modified technique for lapidus procedure. Foot Ankle Clin 2018;23(2):281–95.

11. Tanaka Y, Takakura Y, Sugimoto K, et al. Precise anatomic configuration changes in the first ray of the hallux valgus foot. Foot Ankle Int 2000;21:651–6.

12. Willegger M, Holinka J, Ristl R, et al. Correction power and complications of first tarsometatarsal joint arthrodesis for hallux valgus deformity. Int Orthop 2015; 39(3):467–76.

13. Myerson MS, Badekas A. Hypermobility of the first ray. Foot Ankle Clin 2000;5(3): 469–84.

14. López-López D, Larrainzar-Garijo R, De-Bengoa-Vallejo RB, et al. Effectiveness of the Lapidus plate system in foot surgery: a PRISMA compliant systematic review. Int Wound J 2022;19(3):507–14.

15. Blitz NM, Lee T, Williams K, et al. Early weight bearing after modified lapidus arthodesis: a multicenter review of 80 cases. J Foot Ankle Surg 2010;49(4):357–62.

16. Vieira Cardoso D, Veljkovic A, Wing K, et al. Cohort comparison of radiographic correction and complications between minimal invasive and open lapidus procedures for hallux valgus. Foot Ankle Int 2022;43(10):1277–84.

17. Schmid T, Krause F. The modified Lapidus fusion. Foot Ankle Clin 2014;19(2): 223–33.

18. Lombardi CM, Silhanek AD, Connolly FG, et al. First metatarsocuneiform arthrodesis and Reverdin-Laird osteotomy for treatment of hallux valgus: an intermediate-term retrospective outcomes study. J Foot Ankle Surg 2003;42(2): 77–85.

19. Michels F, Guillo S, de Lavigne C, et al. The arthroscopic Lapidus procedure. Foot Ankle Surg 2011;17(1):25–8.

20. Patel S, Ford LA, Etcheverry J, et al. Modified lapidus arthrodesis: rate of nonunion in 227 cases. J Foot Ankle Surg 2004;43(1):37–42.

21. Wang B, Manchanda K, Lalli T, et al. Identifying risk factors for nonunion of the modified lapidus procedure for the correction of hallux valgus. J Foot Ankle Surg 2022;61(5):1001–6.

22. Lui TH, Chan KB, Ng S. Arthroscopic lapidus arthrodesis. Arthroscopy 2005; 21(12):1516.

23. Vernois J, Redfern D. Lapidus, a percutaneous approach. Foot Ankle Clin 2020; 25(3):407–12.

24. Malagelada F, Sahirad C, Dalmau-Pastor M, et al. Minimally invasive surgery for hallux valgus: a systematic review of current surgical techniques. Int Orthop 2019;43(3):625–37.

25. Yassin M, Bowirat A, Robinson D. Percutaneous surgery of the forefoot compared with open technique - functional results, complications and patient satisfaction. Foot Ankle Surg 2020;26(2):156–216.

26. Blitz NM. New minimally invasive bunion surgery: easier said than done. Foot Ankle Surg: Techn, Rep Cases 2023;3(2).

27. Palmanovich E, Ohana N, Atzmon R, et al. MICA: a learning curve. J Foot Ankle Surg 2020;59(4):781–3.

28. Toepfer A, Strässle M. The percutaneous learning curve of 3rd generation minimally-invasive Chevron and Akin osteotomy (MICA). Foot Ankle Surg 2022 Dec;28(8):1389–98.
29. Chaparro F, Cárdenas PA, Butteri A, et al. Minimally invasive technique with intramedullary nail for treatment of severe hallux valgus: clinical results and surgical technique. J Foot Ankle 2020;14(1):3–8.
30. Leucht AK, Younger A, Veljkovic A, et al. The windswept foot: dealing with metatarsus adductus and toe valgus. Foot Ankle Clin 2020;25(3):413–42.
31. Yeung T, Lui TH. Arthroscopic lapidus arthrodesis of the first tarsometatarsal joint for treatment of hallux valgus deformity of the foot. Arthrosc Tech 2022;11(6).
32. Bean B, Mangold DR, Abousayed M, et al. Percutaneous Modified lapidus procedure with early weightbearing: technique and early outcomes of the first 30 cases. Foot Ankle Orthop 2022;7(1).
33. Baskin ES, Luong K, Aamir A, et al. Identification of portals and evaluation of their safeness for MIS arthrodesis of the 1st tarsometatarsal joint. Foot Ankle Surg: Techn. Rep Cases 2023;3(1).
34. So E, Van Dyke B, McGann MR, et al. Structures at risk from an intermetatarsal screw for Lapidus bunionectomy: a cadaveric study. J Foot Ankle Surg 2019;58(1):62–5.
35. Lehtonen E, Patel H, Lee S, et al. Neurovascular structures at risk with percutaneous fixation in tarsometatarsal fusion: a cadaveric study. Foot 2019;41:19–23.
36. Boffeli TJ, Mahoney KJ. Intraoperative simulated weightbearing lateral foot imaging: the clinical utility and ability to predict sagittal plane position of the first ray in lapidus fusion. J Foot Ankle Surg Off Publ Am Coll Foot Ankle Surg 2016;55(6):1158–63.
37. Ellington JK, Myerson MS, Coetzee JC, et al. The use of the Lapidus procedure for recurrent hallux valgus. Foot Ankle Int 2011;32(7):674–80.
38. Jagadale VS, Thomas RL. A clinicoradiological and functional evaluation of lapidus surgery for moderate to severe bunion deformity shows excellent stable correction and high long-term patient satisfaction. Foot Ankle Spec 2020;13(6):488–93.

Major Heel Reconstructions Through Small Incisions

Klaus Edgar Roth, MD[a],*, Kajetan Klos, MD[b,1], Leif Claassen, MD[c],
Hazibullah Waizy, MD[d]

KEYWORDS

- Minimally invasive surgery • Calcaneal osteotomy • Zadek osteotomy
- Medializing calcaneal osteotomy • Lateralizing calcaneal osteotomy

KEY POINTS

- Minimally invasive calcaneal osteotomies have the same excellent healing potential and deformity correction as open techniques with potentially reduced pain.
- Adhering to safety corridors reduces the risk of injury.
- The release of the periosteum represents a central aspect in achieving a sufficient amount of displacement.
- The learning curve of the procedure is steep.

INTRODUCTION

The position of the hindfoot plays a pivotal role in foot and ankle surgery. It directly affects the distribution of forces between the tibia and heel, thus influencing the load placed on bone, ligaments, and tendons.[1] Calcaneal osteotomies enable adjustments to the calcaneal axis in various planes, which, in the context of correcting deformities, contribute to enhanced foot biomechanics. An offset of 1 cm translation, medial or lateral, creates a significant change in pressure in the ankle joint.[2] Medial displacements unload the lateral joint and increase the load of the medial joint and vice versa in lateral calcaneal displacements.[1] Corrective osteotomies of the calcaneus are therefore powerful surgical tools for realigning the load-bearing axis of the foot and alleviating Achilles tendon tension. They are useful in the form of both medial and

[a] Department of Orthopedic Surgery, Gelenkzentrum Rheinmain, Frankfurter Straße 94, Hochheim 65239, Germany; [b] Department of Orthopedics and Traumatology, University Medical Center of the Johannes Gutenberg University, Mainz, Germany; [c] Department of Trauma, Hand and Reconstructive Surgery, Jena University Hospital, Am Klinikum 1, Jena 07747, Germany; [d] Department of Orthopedics, Orthoprofis, Luisenstrasse 10-11, Hannover 30159, Germany
[1] Present address: Frankfurter Straße 94, Hochheim 65239, Germany.
* Corresponding author. Department of Orthopedic Surgery, Gelenkzentrum Rheinmain, Frankfurter Straße 94, Hochheim 65239, Germany.
E-mail address: e.roth@gelenkzentrum-rheinmain.de

Clin Podiatr Med Surg 42 (2025) 77–87
https://doi.org/10.1016/j.cpm.2024.05.002
0891-8422/25/© 2024 Elsevier Inc. All rights reserved, including those for text and data mining, AI training, and similar technologies.

lateral displacements to treat pes planus and pes cavus, respectively. Calcaneal osteotomies can also be used to treat insertional Achilles tendon disease with asymmetric shortening osteotomy (aka Zadek osteotomy).[1]

Traditionally, calcaneal surgery involved large "open" incisions (Atkins approach) with a lateral approach which carries the risk of wound problems, infections, and neurovascular injuries.[3,4] Over the past several years, surgeons have utilized minimally invasive surgery (MIS) calcaneal osteotomy methods to reduce the rate of wound complications by having smaller incisions and disruption to the soft tissue envelope as whole. Minimally invasive calcaneal osteotomy surgery is made possible by the use of low-speed high-torque rotary burs, which was initially pioneered for bunion surgery by Walker, Redfern, and Vernois.[5,6]

Comparative studies between open/conventional techniques and MIS demonstrate similar outcomes across all aspects of physical function, pain relief, and mobility.[7] MIS offers advantages such as shorter operating times and smaller incisions with comparable radiation exposure.[8] Given these factors, MIS calcaneal osteotomy has gained increasing acceptance.[9]

INDICATIONS

The main indications for MIS calcaneal surgery involve Haglund's deformity, pes planus (flat foot), cavovarus, Haglund's deformity, and Achilles tendinopathy.

Flat Foot

The valgus position of the calcaneus in cases of pes planovalgus is a primary factor contributing to the instability of the lower ankle joint, leading to dissociation of the Chopart joint. Addressing this issue, Gleich[10] introduced a medializing osteotomy with the removal of a medial wedge in 1893 to correct the pes planovalgus deformity.[11] Koutsogiannis[12] later described a technique involving medial and plantar translation through an oblique osteotomy of the calcaneal tuberosity, which has evolved into what is now known as medial displacement calcaneal osteotomy (MDCO). The minimally invasive version is known as minimally invasive medializing calcaneal osteotomy (MIMCO).[8] MIMCO is typically indicated for symptomatic, flexible pes planovalgus and is often performed in conjunction with additional procedures like tendon transfers and reconstructions of the spring ligament complex.[13,14] Contraindications for MIMCO are similar to those for open surgery and include symptomatic arthritis of the subtalar, talonavicular, and calcaneocuboid joints. Cases involving a rigid subtalar joint with limited motion may require a fusion approach. Additionally, in the authors' opinion, large dorsal displacement osteotomies with significant calcaneal inclination are not suitable for minimally invasive techniques and are better managed with open procedures.[8]

Cavovarus Foot

Various osteotomy techniques have been described to address the cavovarus foot deformity.[2,15,16] The Dwyer osteotomy is a common lateralizing procedure that involves a lateral shift combined with a closing wedge osteotomy. Another frequently used approach is the isolated lateralizing calcaneal osteotomy, which is performed through the same lateral approach. Additional superjoint translation of the mobile fragment assists in correcting the cavus deformity.[17] With regard to lateral translations, it has been recommended to limit the displacement to approximately 1 cm to reduce the risk of nerve impingement, tarsal tunnel syndrome, and wound complications.[2]

Various calcaneal osteotomies: Comparative studies, such as one conducted by Krause and colleagues,[18] have shown that various types of calcaneal osteotomies (Dwyer, lateralizing, and Z-type osteotomies) can improve tibiotalar contact pressures and when combined with Dwyer (lateralizing and coronal plane internal rotation), they can achieve optimal correction of varus heel.[2,18,19] The primary goal of these correction approaches is to laterally recenter the Achilles tendon insertion. While flatfoot deformity can often be corrected more easily due to its flexibility, cavovarus deformity is typically more rigid. Consequently, lateralizing osteotomies may be more challenging to displace, necessitating the addition of a bone wedge resection to the procedure.[20]

Many cavovarus feet require arthrodesis more frequently than flatfeet. Therefore, the indications for MIS are significantly narrower and the osteotomies are typically subtractive rather than additive. Optimal position might be achieved with multiple burr passes to attain the desired shift and/or position.[21] The authors encourage practitioners not to settle for smaller translations but to implement the technical recommendations mentioned earlier to achieve precise correction. In some cases, combining a lateral honest shift with lateral rotation may be beneficial.[21]

Achilles Tendinopathy

The treatment of insertional Achilles tendinopathy is a domain of surgical care if conservative therapy fails. The removal of the retrocalcaneal bursitis and the bone prominence/formation, which is referred to as Haglund exostosis, represents an essential pillar of treatment;[22] additional procedures such as Zadek osteotomy are another. The Zadek calcaneal osteotomy, which can be achieved via an MIS approach, tilts the posterior prominence of the calcaneus anteriorly, lowering the posterior prominence of the heel while also elevating the Achilles tendon insertion.[21,23] The Zadek osteotomy consequently reduces the impingement of the Achilles tendon against the calcaneal tuberosity and alters the alignment of the Achilles tendon.[24] Studies that examine the necessary extent of bone subtraction assume a necessary dorsal wedge removal of between 7 and 10 mm.[25] The more horizontal the osteotomy is placed, the more the tension on the Achilles tendon is reduced.[23] The dorsal closing wedge calcaneal osteotomy, whose target sizes are similar to those of the Zadek osteotomy, is placed further dorsally toward the insertion region of the tendon[26] (**Figs. 1–4**).

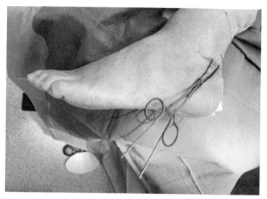

Fig. 1. Insertion of the guide wires and release of the soft tissues with a clamp, marking the osteotomy.

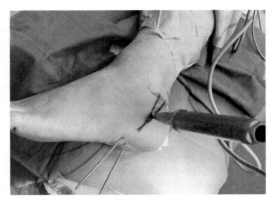

Fig. 2. Insertion of the burr into the lateral cortex and commencing the osteotomy along the guide wires.

Calcaneal osteotomies aim to preserve the tendon attachment to the calcaneal tuberosity; debridement of the tendon itself cannot be achieved with these techniques. However, the extent of damage to the Achilles tendon is the limiting factor of the aforementioned osteotomies. A recent study by Mazura and colleagues[26] in 2022 indicated

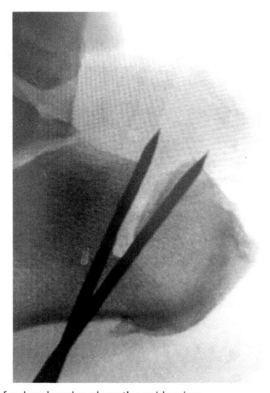

Fig. 3. Removal of a dorsal wedge along the guide wires.

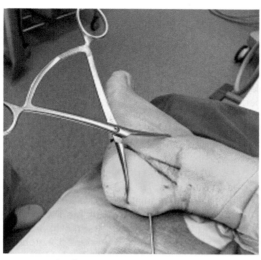

Fig. 4. Closing the osteotomy by forced dorsiflexion and compression with a large clamp.

that more severe degeneration should not be treated without tendon augmentation (eg, flexor hallucis longus transfer).

COMPLICATIONS

Previous studies have indicated wound complications and superficial infections ranging from 0% to 3% in collectives undergoing MIS-MDCO,[3,12,20,27,28] showcase a significant reduction in risk compared to open procedures (3% vs 20%).[3,20] Patients with higher American Society of Anesthesiologists classification (eg, current tobacco use and higher body mass index [BMI]) are identified as having a heightened risk of osteotomy healing complications following minimally invasive MDCO procedures.[27]

The likelihood of delayed bone healing or nonunion is not higher when employing the minimally invasive technique (0%–3%)[27] compared to conventional osteotomies. The theoretic risk of an intraosseous temperature increase can be mitigated by using a burr with chilled irrigation.[29]

Nerve injuries are estimated to occur in 0% to 6% of cases.[3,12,20,27,28] In direct comparisons between open and minimally invasive procedures, the risk of nerve complications with the minimally invasive technique is lower (0%–6% vs 6%–21%).[3,28] If the calcaneus is moved excessively laterally, prophylactic tarsal tunnel release should be considered to offset the tensile stresses generated in this area.[2]

The "safe zone" for minimally invasive calcaneal osteotomy has been identified approximately 1 cm anterior to the line connecting the plantar fascia origin and the posterosuperior apex of the calcaneal tuberosity.[27] A radiographic safe zone was also described by Talusan.[30]

PATIENT POSITIONING AND SURGICAL APPROACH
Patient Positioning

The surgery is carried out in the lateral position. A removable bump under the ipsilateral hip allows internal rotation of the leg if desired.[20] From this position, it is easily possible to transfer the patient onto his back to address the medial structures without losing the sterile cover.[20]

Surgical Approach

To ensure optimal initial conditions and a strictly lateral viewing direction during the procedure, it's important for the medial and lateral talar shoulders to overlap in fluoroscopy. The safe zone, as defined by Talusan,[29] is established by projecting anteriorly 11 mm from a line drawn between the posterosuperior apex of the calcaneus and the origin of the plantar fascia.[20] The direction of the osteotomy is marked on the skin with a sterile pen using a wire under fluoroscopic guidance. An incision approximately 1 cm in length should be made directly in the middle of the tuberosity at the anterior edge of the safe zone,[20] taking the course of the sural nerve into consideration. A clamp is then inserted, and the soft tissue is released along the planned osteotomy.

A 3 mm Shannon burr is brought to the bone surface with the clamp spread, and the lateral cortical bone is perforated (see **Fig. 1**). Under constant irrigation, the unicortical osteotomy is first performed on the cranial lateral cortex, followed by the caudal cortex. While returning the burr to the starting point, the medial cortex is perforated on the medial side with the palpating finger. Parallel to the first-mentioned osteotomies, the mediocranial and mediocaudal cortices are then burred. Lateral and axial images of the calcaneus are checked to ensure proper placement. Minor adjustments in calcaneal length can be made by slightly adjusting the burr's angulation. Anterior angulation leads to greater foreshortening of the calcaneus during medial displacement, while posterior angulation leads to slight lengthening with a medial shift.[20] Optionally, the direction of the osteotomy can be guided using an aid.[20]

To mobilize the tuberosity fragment, a rasp can be passed through the skin incision into the osteotomy to the medial periosteum. Alternatively, a narrow laminar spreader can be used to spread the fragments and aid in parting any remaining periosteal hinge. Release of the periosteum facilitates later translation (**Fig. 5**). In this context, in individual cases of cavovarus, it makes sense to release the medial retinaculum and the periosteum via a separate medial incision.

During the osteotomy

- The ankle should be plantarflexed to relax the Achilles tendon.

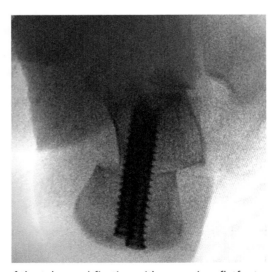

Fig. 5. Translation of the tuber and fixation with screws in a flatfoot.

- For medializing osteotomies, a shift of 8 to 13 mm is typical.
- Lateral shifts are of lower magnitude, typically ranging from 7 to 10 mm.[20]

Fixation

The translation achieved is initially maintained with Kirschner wires (K-wires), whose safe position is verified radiologically. These wires can later serve as a guide for compression screws, which have traditionally been utilized as fixation for calcaneal osteotomies. One or 2 screws measuring 5 to 8 mm are typically sufficient to achieve stability.[15,20,29,31] While screws have proven successful in promoting osseous union, some patients may experience symptomatic apical heel incisions and pain over the screw head, necessitating hardware removal.[20,31] Screw removal may be necessary in up to 20% of cases.[14,20] Although alternative fixation methods, such as lateral step plates and blade plates, have been developed, there is a scarcity of comparative studies available.[32]

The optimal alignment of screws to provide the best stability has not yet been scientifically addressed. Therefore, the author prefers a screw position orthograde to the osteotomy, directed toward the subtalar joint.

While research on the use of K-wires for fixation in MIS-MDCO is lacking, it could present a promising avenue to mitigate hardware-related complications in the future.

Postoperative Care

Calcaneal osteotomies are commonly performed in conjunction with other procedures to correct pes cavus or pes planus deformities. When additional bone surgeries and soft tissue procedures are involved, a rehabilitation timeline of 6 weeks of non-weight-bearing is typically recommended. In rare instances where a calcaneal osteotomy is performed alone or in combination solely with soft tissue procedures, the calcaneus heals rapidly, necessitating only 4 weeks of immobilization with partial weight-bearing. From the author's perspective, the extent of weight-bearing should be determined based on the patient's body weight, with higher BMI prompting caution to avoid dislocation of the osteotomy. However, scientific evidence supporting this approach is currently lacking.

DISCUSSION

MIS for foot and ankle issues has become increasingly popular due to the use of low-speed high-torque burs. Several MIS studies have reported positive outcomes such as smaller scars, reduced postoperative discomfort, quicker recovery, shorter rehabilitation periods, and lower risks of infection and wound complications.[32–34] Durston and colleagues[35] noted that the Shannon bur proves to be a safe, efficient, and time-saving instrument for minimally invasive calcaneal osteotomy.

Kheir and colleagues[4] conducted a retrospective review of 30 cases involving minimally invasive MDCO with 29 cases involving concurrent posterior tibial tendon reconstruction and 1 case addressing a malunited calcaneal fracture. They reported successful clinical union in all cases, without any complications related to wounds or neurovascular issues, and noted appropriate correction of the hindfoot to a neutral position. They described the ease of translating the osteotomy due to the Shannon bur removing approximately 3 mm of bone, which was considered to be more than what a saw would remove. This effectively shortened the heel[32] and facilitated translation. A Brazilian research team presented their findings on 20 cases of cavus correction, utilizing first metatarsal osteotomy and calcaneal osteotomy.[36] They achieved significant correction of the hindfoot with successful healing of all metatarsal osteotomies and no wound complications. However, they reported a 60% rate of sural nerve injury.

In the treatment of Haglund's syndrome, MIS has shown notable advantages over other surgical procedures. A study comparing MIS Zadek osteotomy to alternative methods reported a significant improvement in visual analog scale scores at the 24-month follow-up.[23] The Zadek osteotomy has demonstrated excellent or good outcomes in terms of pain relief, enhancement of daily activities, and improved footwear comfort, achieving a success rate of 75%.[37]

In a study by Kendal and colleagues,[3] MIS procedures using a freehand technique showed a mean displacement of 9.4 mm compared to 10.2 mm in open procedures, along with significantly fewer wound complications and no cases of postoperative neuropathy in the MIS group. Other comparative studies[3,8,28] found no significant differences in clinical outcome scores, radiological union rates, or operative timing between MIS and open procedures, but noted lower rates of wound infections and sural neuropathy in the MIS group.[32]

Minimally invasive techniques can be effectively applied to calcaneal osteotomies, offering the potential for hindfoot correction comparable to open procedures but with less morbidity and pain.[32] They are at least equivalent to open procedures with regard to safety and reliability.[20] Early assessments indicate that MIS calcaneal osteotomy yields comparable patient-reported outcome measure scores in physical function, pain interference, and mobility domains compared to standard open procedures. When proper anatomic landmarks are followed, the risk of neurologic injury is minimized, with some studies suggesting a reduced incidence of lateral calcaneal nerve injury compared to open techniques.[7,20]

In any case, comparative studies[8] did not reveal any notable differences in operating time or exposure to x-rays.

Overall, MIS calcaneal osteotomy is considered a safe alternative to open procedures, offering reliable results with a manageable learning curve, acceptable operating times, and familiar osteosynthesis techniques. However, there is currently a lack of methodologically rigorous evidence to fully support the efficacy of this procedure.

The advent of minimally invasive techniques for correcting calcaneal deformities represents a significant advancement in surgical care. These procedures boast a high success rate, are relatively easy to learn, feature a shallow learning curve, and entail low risk potential. With proper training and the appropriate equipment, surgeons can reliably perform the procedure after a short period of training. Importantly, the extent of translation achieved with minimally invasive techniques is comparable to that of open procedures.

SUMMARY

Minimally invasive calcaneal osteotomy offers potential advantages including reduced postoperative pain, fewer wound complications, less swelling, and a lower risk of iatrogenic injury to neurovascular structures, all while achieving the same correction as open techniques.

CLINICS CARE POINTS

- Precise lateral positioning is crucial as it determines the direction of the osteotomy and ultimately the extent of deformity correction achievable.
- The availability of various burr models is particularly advantageous for subtractive osteotomies.

- Risk factors such as high BMI should be considered when determining the weight-bearing protocol in the patient's postoperative care.
- Although current evidence is lacking, the authors recommend using 2 fixation screws instead of 1, although alternative fixation techniques have not gained widespread acceptance.

DISCLOSURE

The authors have nothing to disclose.

REFERENCES

1. Prat D, Lee W, Charles Farber D. Calcaneal osteotomies. Ann Jt 2020;5.0:29.
2. Steffensmeier SJ, Saltzman CL, Berbaum KS, et al. Effect of medial and lateral displacement calcaneal osteotomies on tibiotalar joint contact stresses. J Orthop Res 1996;14:980–5.
3. Kendal AR, Khalid A, Ball T, et al. Complications of minimally invasive calcaneal osteotomy versus open osteotomy. Foot Ankle Int 2015;36(6):685–90.
4. Kheir E, Borse V, Sharpe J, et al. Medial displacement calcaneal osteotomy using minimally invasive technique. Foot Ankle Int 2015;36(3):248–52.
5. Walker R, Redfern D. Minimally invasive hallux valgus correction: the MICA technique. Orthopaedic Proceedings 2012;94-B(SUPP_XXII):38.
6. Vernois J. The treatment of the hallux valgus with a percutaneous chevron osteotomy. Orthopaedic Proceedings 2011;93-B(SUPP_IV):482.
7. Phillips T, Hall S, Encinas R, et al. Patient reported outcome measures and complication rates after minimally") invasive vs. offene kalkaneusosteotomie. Foot & Ankle Orthopaedics 2023;8(4). 2473011423S00099.
8. Waizy H, Jowett C, Andric V. Minimally invasive versus open calcaneal osteotomies—comparing the intraoperative parameters. Foot 2018;37:113–8.
9. Pang JH, Spalding L, Pasapula C. Minimally invasive surgery: has it come of age? J Orthop Trauma 2023;37(1):62–70.
10. Gleich A. Beitrag zur operativen plattfussbehandlung. Arch Klin Chir 1893;46(1):358–62.
11. Sayres SC, Gu Y, Kiernan S, et al. Comparison of rates of union and hardware removal between large and small cannulated screws for calcaneal osteotomy. Foot Ankle Int 2015;36(1):32–6.
12. Koutsogiannis E. Treatment of mobile flat foot by displacement osteotomy of the calcaneus. J Bone Joint Surg Br 1971;53:96–100.
13. Jowett CRJ, Rodda D, Amin A, et al. Minimally invasive calcaneal osteotomy: a cadaveric and clinical evaluation. Foot Ankle Surg 2016;22(4):244–7.
14. DiDomenico LA, Anain J, Wargo-Dorsey M. Assessment of medial and lateral neurovascular structures after percutaneous posterior calcaneal displacement osteotomy: a cadaver study. J Foot Ankle Surg 2011;50(6):668–71.
15. Dwyer FC. Osteotomy of the calcaneum for pes cavus. J Bone Joint Surg Br 1959;41-B:80–6.
16. Dwyer FC. The present status of the problem of pes cavus. Clin Orthop Relat Res 1975;106:254–75.
17. Bariteau JT, Blankenhorn BD, Tofte JN, et al. What is the role and limit of calcaneal osteotomy in the cavovarus foot? Foot Ankle Clin 2013;18:697–714.

18. Krause FG, Sutter D, Waehnert D, et al. Ankle joint pressure changes in a pes cavovarus model after lateralizing calcaneal osteotomies. Foot Ankle Int 2010; 31:741–6.
19. An TW, Michalski M, Jansson K, et al. Comparison of lateralizing calcaneal osteotomies for varus hindfoot correction. Foot Ankle Int 2018;39:1229–36.
20. Guyton GP. Minimally invasive osteotomies of the calcaneus. Foot Ankle Clin 2016;21(3):551–66.
21. Karaismailoglu Bedri, Nassour N, Duggan J, et al. Effect of sequential burr passes on osteotomy magnitude and calcaneal morphology in minimally invasive Zadek osteotomy. Foot Ankle Surg 2023.
22. Chen Jie, Janney CF, Khalid MA, et al. Management of insertional Achilles tendinopathy. J Am Acad Orthop Surg 2022;30(10):e751–9.
23. Poutoglidou F, Drummond I, Patel A, et al. Clinical outcomes and complications of the Zadek calcaneal osteotomy in insertional Achilles tendinopathy: a systematic review and meta-analysis: level of evidence II. Foot Ankle Surg 2023.
24. Boffeli TJ, Peterson MC. The Keck and Kelly wedge calcaneal osteotomy for Haglund's deformity: a technique for reproducible results. J Foot Ankle Surg 2012; 51(3):398–401.
25. Tourne Y, Baray AL, Barthelemy R, et al. The Zadek calcaneal osteotomy in Haglund's syndrome of the heel: clinical results and a radiographic analysis to explain its efficacy. Foot Ankle Surg 2022;28(1):79–87.
26. Mazura M, Goldman T, Stanislav P Jr, et al. Calcaneal osteotomy due to insertional calcaneal tendinopathy: preoperative planning. J Orthop Surg Res 2022; 17(1):478.
27. Coleman MM, Abousayed MM, Thompson JM, et al. Risk factors for complications associated with minimally invasive medial displacement calcaneal osteotomy. Foot Ankle Int 2021;42(2):121–31.
28. Gutteck N, Zeh A, Wohlrab D, et al. Comparative results of percutaneous calcaneal osteotomy in correction of hindfoot deformities. Foot Ankle Int 2019;40(3): 276–81.
29. Reddy SC, Schipper ON, Li J. The effect of chilled vs room-temperature irrigation on thermal energy dissipation during minimally invasive calcaneal osteotomy of cadaver specimens. Foot & Ankle Orthopaedics 2022;7(4). 2473011422113 6548.
30. Talusan PG, Cata E, Tan EW, et al. Safe zone for neural structures in medial displacement calcaneal osteotomy: a cadaveric and radiographic investigation. Foot Ankle Int 2015;36(12):1493–8.
31. Johnson KA, Strom DE. Tibialis posterior tendon dysfunction. Clin Orthop Relat Res 1989;239:196–206, 1976-2007).
32. Sherman Thomas I, Gregory P Guyton. Minimal incision/minimally invasive medializing displacement calcaneal osteotomy. Foot Ankle Int 2018;39(1):119–28.
33. Choi Jun Young, Jin Soo Suh. A novel technique of minimally invasive calcaneal osteotomy for intractable insertional Achilles tendinopathy associated with Haglund deformity. Foot Ankle Surg 2022;28(5):578–83.
34. Vaggi S, Vitali F, Zanirato A, et al. Minimally invasive surgery in medial displacement calcaneal osteotomy for acquired flatfoot deformity: a systematic review of the literature. Arch Orthop Trauma Surg 2024;144(3):1139–47.
35. Durston Abigail, Bahoo R, Kadambande S, et al. Minimally invasive calcaneal osteotomy: does the Shannon burr endanger the neurovascular structures? A cadaveric study. J Foot Ankle Surg 2015;54(6):1062–6.

36. Astolfi RS, de Vasconcelos Coelho JV, Ribeiro HCT, et al. Cavus foot correction using a full percutaneous procedure: a case series. Int J Environ Res Publ Health 2021;18(19):10089.
37. Nordio A, Chan JJ, Guzman JZ, et al. Percutaneous Zadek osteotomy for the treatment of insertional Achilles tendinopathy. Foot Ankle Surg 2020;26(7): 818–21.

Where Small Incision Fusions of the Foot Work Wonders

Brian G. Loder, DPM

KEYWORDS

- Arthrodesis • Minimal incision • Percutaneous • Arthritis

KEY POINTS

- Discuss the role of arthrodesis of different joints in the foot.
- Discuss the use of percutaneous arthrodesis in the foot.
- Discuss the indications for percutaneous arthrodesis of various joints in the foot.
- Provide tips and pearls for the percutaneous arthrodesis of various joints in the foot.
- Discuss the post-surgical protocol of percutaneous arthrodesis of various joints in the foot including risks and postoperative complications.

INTRODUCTION

Multiple pathologies in the foot and ankle are treated with joint arthrodesis, which include: realignment of deformities, stabilization of soft tissue imbalance, treatment of post-traumatic and inflammatory arthritis, as well as treatment for neuromuscular disorders. Arthrodesis can be the sole procedure like when used for isolated first metatarsophalangeal joint for hallux rigidus, combined with other procedures like a talonavicular arthrodesis when used for progressive flat foot deformity or multiple joint arthrodesis like seen in medial column arthrodesis or a triple arthrodesis.[1–20] Arthrodesis, whether primary or when combined with other procedures, has a long convalescence stage that results in atrophy and muscle weakness. Complications associated with arthrodesis include malunion, non-union, and adjacent joint arthrosis.[21–23]

The percutaneous approach to foot pathology has experienced resurgence in the last decade. Originally used for hallux valgus correction or removal of prominent bone spurs, percutaneous surgery has been gaining popularity for primary arthrodesis in the foot. The advantages of the percutaneous approach over the open approach included less edema, smaller scars, lower risk of infection, and reduce operating room time.[24–26] When a surgeon chooses to perform an arthrodesis through a

Michigan Minimal Invasive and Reconstructive Foot and Ankle Fellowship, 15760 19 Mile Road, Suite E, Clinton Township, MI 48038, USA
E-mail address: bloder@detroitfa.com

Clin Podiatr Med Surg 42 (2025) 89–101
https://doi.org/10.1016/j.cpm.2024.05.003
0891-8422/25/© 2024 Elsevier Inc. All rights are reserved, including those for text and data mining, AI training, and similar technologies.
podiatric.theclinics.com

percutaneous incision, they lose control of visualization and are forced to rely on feel to ensure all the cartilaginous surface has been resected. The importance of adequate joint preparation cannot be overstated and there must be a balance between adequate removal of articular surface and minimal bone loss so as not to require large amounts of bone graft.[27] Surgeons new to a minimally invasive surgery (MIS) should be aware that any percutaneous arthrodesis should be converted to an open procedure when the surgeon feels the outcome will be compromised through the percutaneous approach. As a surgeon becomes more comfortable with the percutaneous approach, this conversion should become less common. Another limitation with the percutaneous approach is the limitation of fixation options. With open procedures the surgeon has more options available like plates, staples, and the combination of those with the additions of screws. Percutaneous arthrodesis does limit the surgeon to percutaneous fixation, which may at first require more confidence and experience to perform. Finally, percutaneous arthrodesis is not without its complications, these include iatrogenic nerve injury, inadequate joint preparation, and inadequate fixation, which may lead to delayed or nonunion, as well as malunion.

Operating Room Set-up and Patient Positioning

Although the operating room set-up and patient positioning has variability, novice surgeons are encouraged to use a standard approach so they may develop a reproducible learning curve. I prefer to perform all percutaneous surgery in the same way, to rely as much as possible on muscle memory. I position the patient bed slightly more to the back of the operating room; this allows enough space for the mini fluoroscopy at the foot of the bed. Since I am right-handed, I always sit to the left of the patient whether I am operating on either limb. If I am operating on the right limb, I will position the left limb out of my way using a knee bolster (**Fig. 1**). No limb adjustment is required if I am operating on the left limb. The patient is positioned in such a way that the feet are hanging off the end of the bed approximately 12 inches. This allows the appropriate foot to be in contact with the fluoroscopy throughout the entire procedure (**Fig. 2**). The use of a pneumatic tourniquet is unnecessary; the active bleeding reduces the heat generated from the bur. The foot pedal for the fluoroscopy and the power source are used in tandem while actively using both the right and left foot. Full lead armor is recommended to reduce exposure from repetitive fluoroscopy use. Instrumentation is minimal and includes only those instruments created to work in percutaneous incisions (**Fig. 3**). It is important to allow adequate surgical time when first adopting the percutaneous technique, although reduced times are a benefit of the percutaneous, this is only seen later in the learning process.

MINIMALLY INVASIVE SURGERY HALLUX INTERPHALANGEAL ARTHRODESIS

Angular and arthritic deformities of the great toe are well-suited for the percutaneous approach. Open procedures can cause painful scars in shoe gear that the percutaneous can avoid. The technique for an MIS hallux interphalangeal arthrodesis is sequenced in **Fig. 4**. A medial midline incision or approach is recommended. A freer is placed into the joint and confirmed under fluoroscopy. A bur is introduced into the incision and the articular cartilage is removed carefully from the adjacent articular surfaces under fluoroscopic guidance. Slightly more bone can be removed in instances of a long great toe. Once adequate resection is achieved, the bur is removed, and a rasp is used to remove any articular remnants. Copious irrigation is performed to ensure adequate clearance of any bone particles that remain. Provisional fixation is used to ensure the desired alignment; I utilize the artificial floor technique to simulate

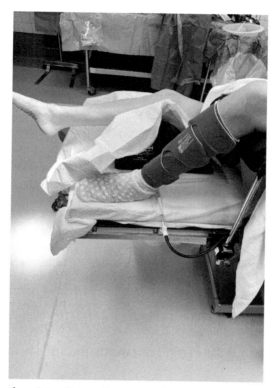

Fig. 1. Positioning of a minimally invasive surgery (MIS) patient.

weight-bearing position.[28] Once the desired alignment is achieved, I use 2 crossing headless compression screws from distal to proximal, 1 medial and 1 lateral for stable fixation. An alternative option is 1 screw axial down the tip of the toe distal to proximal, although this can allow rotation to occur. My postoperative ambulator protocol is to allow for immediate weight-bearing in a stiff sole surgical shoe postoperatively

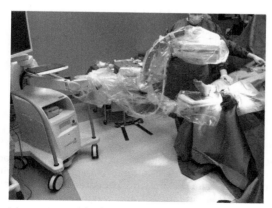

Fig. 2. Patient's foot in contact with Fluoroscopy unit.

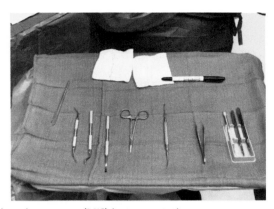

Fig. 3. Minimally invasive surgery (MIS) instrumentation.

for the first 4 weeks. At postoperative week 5, the operative foot is placed in a stiff athletic shoe or sandal. The return to physical activity is tempered by the findings seen on serial radiographs. Full consolidation occurs at 12 to 16 weeks. Complications associated with this procedure are minimal but include hallucal nerve irritation, malunion, and non-union, which are all iatrogenic issues that can occur with poor surgical technique.

MINIMALLY INVASIVE SURGERY FIRST METATARSOPHALANGEAL JOINT ARTHRODESIS

The first metatarsophalangeal joint (MPJ) is the most common arthritic joint in the foot. Heine reported that it was only second in disability to the knee.[29] Howard and colleagues reviewed 517 consecutive radiographs of adult patients being seen for acute trauma to the foot and found that the radiographic evidence of osteoarthritis of the first MPJ was 25%.[30] The First MPJ arthrodesis is a common procedure for both hallux valgus and hallux rigidus. The open surgical procedure for first MPJ arthrodesis does carry some frequent complications including painful cicatrix, irritable hardware,

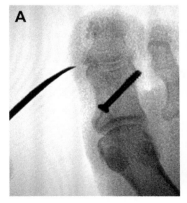
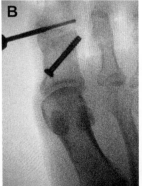
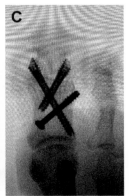

Fig. 4. (*A*) Elevator is used to identify the location of the joint to be fused. (*B*) Bur is placed into the hallux interphalangeal joint. (*C*) Crossing screws fixation.

and non-union.[31] The percutaneous first MPJ arthrodesis may mitigate some of these risks and an alternative approach.

The percutaneous first MPJ arthrodesis can be approached through the medial or dorsal approach. I use the medial approach with a dorsal lateral utility incision if needed. The procedure is performed through a 1 cm incision at the level of the joint; a freer is inserted in the joint to define the working space. A 3.1 wedge bur is used to remove the articular surface from the base of the proximal phalange and then the head of metatarsal is removed in an equivalent manner. This approach creates planar surfaces and requires keeping mindfulness of all planes when performing the resection. If conical surfaces are desired, then a dorsal medial and dorsal lateral approach are required to fashion the surfaces. I have not found any difference in the outcomes or functional length of the first ray. Once the surfaces are prepared, a rasp or curette can be used to evaluate the resected surfaces. This technique is common in percutaneous surgery and getting the feel of an articular surface versus an osseous surface is mandatory to ensure appropriate cartilage removal. At this point, the desired position is ensured, and provisional fixation is performed. The artificial floor technique is used to ensure appropriate position of the great toe in relation to the weight-bearing surface. I use 2 crossing headless compression screws, 1 distal medial and 1 proximal medial (**Fig. 5**). The incisions are reapproximated with 4-0 Nylon and a soft compression dressing is applied. My postoperative ambulatory protocol (not studied) is to permit the patient to ambulate in a flat orthopedic shoe for 4 weeks and then it is

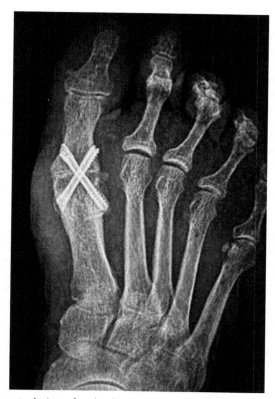

Fig. 5. Crossed screw technique for the first metatarsophalangeal joint.

converted to a stiff sole athletic shoe at the fifth week. Radiographs are taken in weeks 2, 8, and 14. Full return to all activities happens when radiograph confirms full consolidation.

When comparing outcomes of the open versus percutaneous approach for first MPJ fusions, in my hands, I have seen less swelling, less pain, quicker return to normal shoes, and far less hardware irritation from the percutaneous approach. In some cases, there will be a large dorsal osteophyte associated with the hallux rigidus. In these cases, the incision for the proximal medial screw can be used to perform a resection in the standard percutaneous Cheilectomy approach.

MINIMALLY INVASIVE SURGERY TARSOMETATARSAL ARTHRODESIS

The tarsometatarsal joint complex, also known as the Lisfranc joint named by the Napoleonic era field surgeon Jacques Lisfranc, is a combination of osseous, capsular, and ligament structures that define the division of the forefoot and midfoot.[32,33] The Lisfranc joint has been a focus of pathology more recently due to increased awareness of acute injury and its attribute to the development of hallux valgus development. The involvement of the first tarsometatarsal joint in the development of hallux valgus has been debated in literature recently.[34] Correction of hallux valgus with first tarsometatarsal joint arthrodesis is commonly performed.[35–38] The utilization of tarsometatarsal arthrodesis is not limited to the first metatarsal medial cuneiform joint. Of the 3 columns of the tarsometatarsal joint, the central column is most often involved in painful arthritic conditions.[39] When conservative measures fail, isolated or combined arthrodesis of the central column has been utilized to alleviate pain.[40] The open approach to the central column can be a little more difficult given the proximity of the dorsal neurovascular structures. Medial column arthrodesis whether in-situ or combined with angular correction is well-suited for a percutaneous approach. A medial percutaneous incision is the best approach to the joint since it avoids the medial dorsal cutaneous nerve and the vital tendinous structures.[41] A technician's tip is to place K-wires on each side of the articular cartilage to act as guard rails and to help reduce shortening.[42] An external joint distractor may be used to help create joint space when first approaching the joint with the bur, if the joint is hypermobile then the external distractors should be unnecessary (**Fig. 6**). Fixation is achieved with 2 crossing headless cannulated screws and a third screw can be used to stabilize the medial column to the central column.

Central column arthrodesis may be even more amendable to percutaneous arthrodesis than the medial column. The avoidance of a painful dorsal scar may be the primary reason to perform the fusion through a percutaneous approach. The second and third tarsometatarsal joints can either be approached through a singular dorsal incision placed equally between the 2 joint surfaces, or they can be approached through separate incisions. Excessive resection should be avoided as it will make apposition difficult and require the need for bone grafting. Fixation can be achieved with a single or double headless compression screw from distal to proximal for each joint (**Fig. 7**). Postoperation, my patients are placed in a non-weight-bearing posterior splint for the initial 2 weeks. After suture removal, I place a controlled ankle motion (CAM) boot for 4 weeks and encouraged to progress to full weight-bearing as tolerated. The patient should transition to athletic shoe gear at 8 to 10 weeks postoperatively. Postoperative complications include painful cicatrix, delayed or nonunion, and malunion, which have been less significant in the percutaneous approach when compared to the open approach in my experience with my patient population.

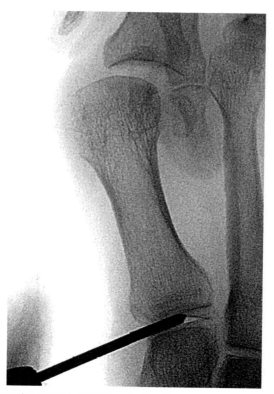

Fig. 6. Minimally invasive surgery (MIS) bur in the first tarsometatarsal joint. (Image Courtesy of Holly Johnson MD.)

MINIMALLY INVASIVE SURGERY MIDTARSAL (CHOPART'S) ARTHRODESIS

The midtarsal joint (Chopart's) complex is the division of the midfoot and rearfoot and consists of the talonavicular and calcaneocuboid joints and their stabilizing ligaments.[43–45] The epidemiology of Chopart's injuries is poorly understood and under-reported, the incidence is 4 out of 100,000 person per year.[46] Most Chopart's injuries are treated with reduction and stabilization; primary arthrodesis is reserved for those cases that have large loss of articular surfaces. Primary arthrodesis of the Chopart's or its parts is commonly seen as treatment for the painful pronated foot, progressive collapsing foot deformity, or in degenerating arthritis like seen in post-traumatic or rheumatoid arthritis. The talonavicular joint is often fused in advance rearfoot pathology, the joint can be an isolated fusion, combined with the subtalar joint in a medial double, or combined with the subtalar and calcaneocuboid joint like seen in a triple arthrodesis.[7,14,16,47] In all scenarios, the talonavicular joint is well-suited to be approached percutaneously. I approach the talonavicular joint through a dorsal medial approach for the medial and central joint access and will sometimes utilize a lateral incision if the lateral articular surface is difficult to access. Due to the shape of the joint, I recommend joint distraction with either an external joint distractor or a laminar spreader (**Fig. 8**A). The talar articular surface should be approached first and the convexity should be preserved as much as possible. Once the articular surface has been removed, there will be adequate working space to remove the navicular articular. A curette or rasp will

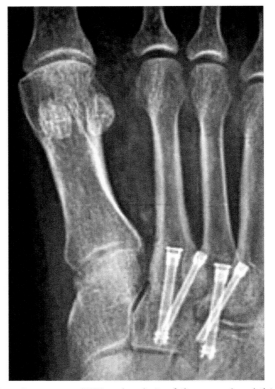

Fig. 7. Minimally invasive surgery (MIS) arthrodesis of the second and third tarsometatarsal joints.

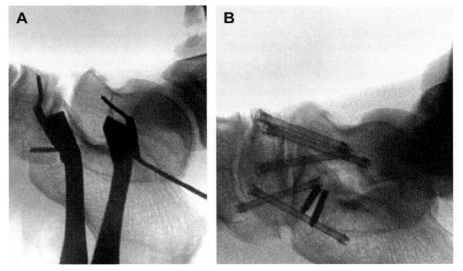

Fig. 8. (*A*) An external joint spreader used to distract the talonavicular joint. (*B*) Percutaneous fixation of a midtarsal arthrodesis.

allow the assessment of appropriate articular removal. I also recommend subchondral drilling of both resected surfaces. Maintaining the concavity of the joint allows for a more precise correction because it can be dialed in once the patient's reaction is complete. If too much bone is removed, a percutaneous bone graft from the lateral calcaneus or allogenic bone graft can be used to fill the void. I prefer 2 to 3 percutaneous screws from the navicular to the talar head for fixation. I will use a chamfered compression screw to reduce dorsal irritation (**Fig. 8**B). A benefit to the percutaneous approach to the talonavicular joint is that ligamentotaxis is preserved and the joint is much more stable than it otherwise would be with the open procedure.

The calcaneocuboid joint is a much easier joint for the percutaneous approach than the talonavicular joint. The saddle joint surface allows a direct approach. I will still use osseous external retraction when resecting the surfaces; this does prevent excessive bone removal. Depending on the deformity and collapse of the joint surface, bone graft may be necessary. Although the percutaneous incision needs to be made larger to facilitate the insertion of the bone graft, the incisions are still much smaller than those created for the open procedure. My fixation of choice is 2 crossing compression screws, one from the anterior talar process and the other from the dorsal lateral cuboid.

Percutaneous arthrodesis of the midfoot requires non weight-bearing for 4 to 6 weeks and then weight-bearing for 2 to 4 weeks in a CAM boot. I have found sequential radiographs are helpful to start weight-bearing as early as possible. I have been able to start weight-bearing in most of my patient population at 4 weeks. Percutaneous talonavicular arthrodesis can incorporate the navicular cuneiform joints as well if midfoot collapse present. The approach to the navicular cuneiform joints is remarkable like the midtarsal joints; the use of bone graft is far more common in this area due to the difficulty of approximating the joint surfaces. The argument of the total accumulation of all the percutaneous incisions can add up to the length of the 1 incision is debatable, but the reduction in dissection and the preservation of the soft tissue envelope with the percutaneous approach cannot be overstated.

MINIMALLY INVASIVE SURGERY SUBTALAR ARTHRODESIS

The subtalar arthrodesis is a vital procedure used in the treatment of post-traumatic osteoarthritis, progressing collapsing flat foot and inflammatory arthropathies.[48–50] The open procedure has been a workhorse for the foot and ankle surgeon for years with dependable outcomes and minimal risk. In-situ arthrodesis has better reported outcome than the distraction arthrodesis used for ill-reduced calcaneal fractures.[51] Arthroscopic arthrodesis of the subtalar joint has gained popularity over the years with experienced arthroscopists.[52–54] Recently, some minimally invasive surgeons have abandoned the bulky arthroscopic approach for the slimmed down minimally invasive approach. Although there are some surgeons are using a hybrid approach, which utilized the quicker and more invasive MIS bur equipment for joint resection but are still inserting the arthroscope to ensure complete cartilaginous resection. The percutaneous and arthroscopic techniques use the sinus tarsi and posterior lateral approach to access the entire posterior subtalar joint surface. The need to prep the middle and anterior facets are still up for debate. I encourage all novice surgeons to not fully be comfortable with the blind assessment described in this article but to utilize the arthroscopic approach to ensure adequate articular surface removal. Minor angular corrections are not a contraindication to the percutaneous approach, but distraction arthrodesis requires the open procedure. The use of autogenic or allogenic bone graft can enhance the fusions in certain populations. Fixation of choice for

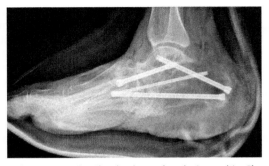

Fig. 9. Minimally invasive surgery (MIS) subtalar arthrodesis used in Charcot reconstruction.

me is 1 or 2 headless screws from the plantar posterior heel in the talus body (**Fig. 9**). Post-operatively, a bulky posterior splint is used for 2-week non weight-bearing. After suture removal, I maintain non weight-bearing in a CAM boot and encourage range-of-motion exercises for 4 more weeks. After serial radiographs confirm consolidation, weight-bearing at 6 weeks in the CAM boot is permitted. Overall I have found less incisional pain and less sural nerve risk with the percutaneous approach.

SUMMARY

Traditional arthrodesis of the joints of the foot has been met with varying degrees of success due to the risk of non-union, neuroma formation, and incisional complications. The resurgence of minimal invasive techniques in the foot and ankle has brought about a host of innovative approaches in the foot and ankle that may mitigate some of these obstacles. The ability to fuse a joint while maintaining ligamentotaxis and a soft tissue envelope has given the percutaneous approach a slight upper hand. The fact that percutaneous techniques have been slow to be adopted, have more to do with the lack of technical skill set than quality of outcomes. Quality peer review studies on the outcomes of percutaneous arthrodesis of the foot have been rare in the literature, but as more individuals adopt the technique, the increase in patient reported outcomes and validated studies should throw better light on its benefits when compared to the open procedure. I encourage the reader to start slowly in the process of gaining a skill set. Utilizing less complicated approaches to develop the appropriate "bur feel" will help the novice surgeon build confidence. I cannot overstate the benefits of a well-structured cadaveric training program prior to embarking on the road to minimally invasive foot surgery. The presence of this edition can be proof enough that minimally-invasive foot surgery is not just a fad but is here to stay. I hope the insights in this article assist you in advancing your percutaneous techniques to arthrodesis of the joints of the foot.

CLINICS CARE POINTS

- The use of percutaneous techniques is expanding in the foot and ankle.
- In-situ arthrodesis of the small joints of the foot and ankle are ideal for percutaneous approach.
- The surgeon develop the appropriate feel and confidence in using a bur through a percutaneous approach

DISCLOSURE

Enovis - consultant/Design. Treace-Consultant/Design; GLW- investor.

REFERENCES

1. Aziz S, Jones A, Bhatia M. A qualitative study of the functional outcomes following first metatarsophalangeal joint (MTPJ) arthrodesis based on a procedure focused questionnaire. Journal of Foot & Ankle Surgery 2022;61(6):1182–6.
2. Crowell A, Van J, Meyr A. Early weight-bearing after arthrodesis of the first metatarsal-phalangeal joint: a systematic review of the incidence of non-union. J Foot and Ankle Surg 2018;57(6):1200–3.
3. Donegan R, Blume P. Functional results and patient satisfaction of first metatarsophalangeal joint arthrodesis using dual crossed screw fixation. J Foot Ankle Surg 2017;56(2):291–7.
4. Guo H, et al. A modified foot and ankle score for assessing patient outcomes after first metatarsophalangeal arthrodesis. J Foot & Ankle Surg 2018;57(2):254–8.
5. Stevens J, et al. Clinical outcome following total joint replacement and arthrodesis for hallux rigidus: a Systematic review. JBJS Reviews 2017;5(11):e2.
6. Coulon, Geraldo de, Turcot K, Canavese F, et al. Talonavicular arthrodesis for the treatment of neurological flat foot deformity in pediatric patients: clinical and radiographic evaluation of 29 feet. J Pediatr Orthop 2011;31(5):557–63.
7. Fischer S, Oepping J, Altmeppen J, et al. Adult-Acquired flatfoot deformity: combined talonavicular arthrodesis and calcaneal displacement osteotomy versus double arthrodesis. J Clin Med 2022;11(3).
8. Harper MC. Talonavicular arthrodesis for the acquired flatfoot in the adult. Clin Orthop Relat Res 1999;(365):65–8.
9. Harper MC, Tisdel CL. Talonavicular arthrodesis for the painful adult acquired flatfoot. Foot Ankle Int 1996;17(11):658–61.
10. Lendrum JA, Hunt KJ. Medial column fusions in flatfoot deformities: naviculocuneiform and talonavicular. Foot Ankle Clin 2022;27(4):769–86.
11. Mothershed RA, Stapp MD, Smith TF. Talonavicular arthrodesis for correction of posterior tibial tendon dysfunction. Clin Podiatr Med Surg 1999;16(3):501–26.
12. Naldo JV, Kugach K. Naviculocuneiform arthrodesis for treatment of adult-acquired flatfoot deformity. Clin Podiatr Med Surg 2023;40(2):293–305.
13. Ramírez-Barragán A, et al. Long-term outcomes of talonavicular arthrodesis for the treatment of Planovalgus foot in Children with Cerebral Palsy. J Pediatr Orthop 2022;42(4):e377–83.
14. Weinraub GM, Heilala MA. Isolated talonavicular arthrodesis for adult onset flatfoot deformity/posterior tibial tendon dysfunction. Clin Podiatr Med Surg 2007;24(4):745–52, ix.
15. Cates NK, et al. Double versus triple arthrodesis fusion rates: a systematic review. J Foot Ankle Surg 2022;61(4):907–13.
16. D'Angelantonio AM, Schick FA, Arjomandi N. Triple arthrodesis. Clin Podiatr Med Surg 2012;29(1):91–102.
17. Knupp M, Stufkens SA, Hintermann B. Triple arthrodesis. Foot Ankle Clin 2011;16(1):61–7.
18. Madi NS, Fletcher AN, Easley ME. Double and triple tarsal fusions in the severe rigid flatfoot deformity. Foot Ankle Clin 2022;27(4):805–18.
19. McCormick JJ, Johnson JE. Medial column procedures in the correction of adult acquired flatfoot deformity. Foot Ankle Clin 2012;17(2):283–98.

20. Schleunes S, Catanzariti A. Addressing medial column instability in flatfoot deformity. Clin Podiatr Med Surg 2023;40(2):271–91.
21. Cardoso DV, Veljkovic A. General considerations about foot and ankle arthrodesis. Any way to improve our results? Foot Ankle Clin 2022;27(4):701–22.
22. Murphy LJ, Mendicino RW, Catanzariti AR. Revisional hindfoot arthrodesis. Clin Podiatr Med Surg 2009;26(1):59–78.
23. Vier D, Ellington JK. Persistent pain after hindfoot fusion. Foot Ankle Clin 2022; 27(2):327–41.
24. Bauer T. Percutaneous hindfoot and midfoot fusion. Foot Ankle Clin 2016;21(3): 629–40.
25. Schipper ON, et al. Percutaneous techniques in orthopedic foot and ankle surgery. Orthop Clin North Am 2020;51(3):403–22.
26. Stiglitz Y, Cazeau C. Minimally invasive surgery and percutaneous surgery of the hindfoot and midfoot. Eur J Orthop Surg Traumatol 2018;28(5):839–47.
27. Zhao JZ, Kaiser PB, DeGruccio C, et al. Quality of MIS vs open joint preparations of the foot and ankle. Foot Ankle Int 2022;43(7):948–56.
28. Strony J, Rascoe AS, Marcus RE. Validation of the artificial floor technique in first metatarsophalangeal joint arthrodesis. Clin Orthop Relat Res 2022;480(10):2002–9.
29. Heine J. Über die Arthritis deformans. Virchows Arch Pathol Anat Physiol Klin Med 1926;260(3):521–663.
30. Howard N, Cowen C, Caplan M, et al. Radiological prevalence of degenerative arthritis of the first metatarsophalangeal joint. Foot Ankle Int 2014;35(12):1277–81.
31. Sebag JA, et al. The first metatarsophalangeal joint: updates on revision arthrodesis and malunions. Clin Podiatr Med Surg 2023;40(4):569–80.
32. DiDomenico LA, Cross D. Tarsometatarsal/Lisfranc joint. Clin Podiatr Med Surg 2012;29(2):221–42, vii-viii.
33. Pearce CJ, Calder JD. Surgical anatomy of the midfoot. Knee Surg Sports Traumatol Arthrosc 2010;18(5):581–6.
34. Mansur NSB, de Souza Nery CA. Hypermobility in hallux valgus. Foot Ankle Clin 2020;25(1):1–17.
35. Santrock RD, Smith B. Hallux valgus deformity and treatment: a three-dimensional approach: modified technique for lapidus procedure. Foot Ankle Clin 2018;23(2):281–95.
36. Dujela MD, Langan T, Cottom JM, et al. Lapidus arthrodesis. Clin Podiatr Med Surg 2022;39(2):187–206.
37. Do DH, Sun JJ, Wukich DK. Modified lapidus procedure and hallux valgus: a systematic review and update on triplanar correction. Orthop Clin North Am 2022; 53(4):499–508.
38. Reilly ME, Conti MS, Day J, et al. Modified lapidus vs scarf osteotomy outcomes for treatment of hallux valgus deformity. Foot Ankle Int 2021;42(11):1454–62.
39. Riehl J, Tomaszewski D, Cush G. Midfoot arthritis: evaluation and treatment, surgical and nonsurgical. Current Orthopaedic Practice 2008;19(3):249–52.
40. Seybold J, Coetzee J. Surgical management of posttraumatic midfoot deformity and arthritis. Tech Foot Ankle Surg 2016;15:79–86, 2.
41. Boffeli T, Gervais S. Accuracy of palpation to identify the medial branch of the medial dorsal cutaneous nerve in medial column surgery: correlation of preoperative nerve marking with intraoperative findings during lapidus fusion. J Foot & Ankle Surg 2021;60(1):2–5.
42. Vernois J, Redfern D, GRECMIP soon MIFAS. Lapidus, a percutaneous approach. Foot Ankle Clin 2020;25(3):407–12.

43. Tweed JL, Campbell JA, Thompson RJ, et al. The function of the midtarsal joint: a review of the literature. Foot 2008;18(2):106–12.
44. Walter WR, et al. Imaging of Chopart (midtarsal) joint complex: normal anatomy and posttraumatic findings. AJR Am J Roentgenol 2018;211(2):416–25.
45. Walter WR, et al. Normal anatomy and traumatic injury of the midtarsal (Chopart) joint complex: an imaging primer. Radiographics 2019;39(1):136–52.
46. Ponkilainen VT, Laine HJ, Mäenpää HM, et al. Incidence and characteristics of midfoot injuries. Foot Ankle Int 2019;40(1):105–12.
47. Philippot R, Wegrzyn J, Besse JL. Arthrodesis of the subtalar and talonavicular joints through a medial surgical approach: a series of 15 cases. Arch Orthop Trauma Surg 2010;130(5):599–603.
48. Davies MB, Rosenfeld PF, Stavrou P, et al. A comprehensive review of subtalar arthrodesis. Foot Ankle Int 2007;28(3):295–7.
49. Yildirim T, Sofu H, Çamurcu Y, et al. Isolated subtalar arthrodesis. Acta Orthop Belg 2015;81(1):155–60.
50. Wirth SH, Zimmermann SM, Viehöfer AF. Open technique for in situ subtalar fusion. Foot Ankle Clin 2018;23(3):461–74.
51. Chraim M, Recheis S, Alrabai H, et al. Midterm outcome of subtalar joint revision arthrodesis. Foot Ankle Int 2021;42(7):824–32.
52. Walter RP, Walker RW, Butler M, et al. Arthroscopic subtalar arthrodesis through the sinus tarsi portal approach: a series of 77 cases. Foot Ankle Surg 2018;24(5):417–22.
53. Coulomb R, et al. Do clinical results of arthroscopic subtalar arthrodesis correlate with CT fusion ratio? Orthop Traumatol Surg Res 2019;105(6):1125–9.
54. Wagner E, Melo R. Subtalar arthroscopic fusion. Foot Ankle Clin 2018;23(3):475–83.

A New Paradigm for Failed Bunions with Minimally Invasive Methods

David T. Wong, DPM

KEYWORDS

- Revision bunion surgery • Minimally invasive bunion surgery • MIBS
- Failed bunion surgery

KEY POINTS

- Failed bunion surgeries have traditionally been addressed through open surgical techniques, which involve procedures such as soft tissue balancing, osteotomies with internal fixation, and fusions of the first metatarsophalangeal joint (MPJ) and first tarsometatarsal joint (TMTJ).
- Modern percutaneous and minimally invasive approaches have gained traction in orthopedic practice for various procedures, including revising failed bunion surgeries.
- These newer minimally invasive techniques offer several advantages over open procedures, including: quicker recovery times, reduced operating room duration, minimal scarring, effective correction of deformities, and the ability for early weight-bearing, as highlighted in recent studies.
- This approach is versatile and can be effectively applied to a wide range of failed bunion deformities, leading to improved patient outcomes.

INTRODUCTION

Hallux valgus (bunion) is a common painful big toe joint subluxation deformity characterized by lateral displacement of the great toe and a noticeable medial bony prominence of the first metatarsophalangeal joint (MPJ). There are numerous surgical methods to treat bunions without a true consensus on the best or most effective surgical solution (**Table 1**).[1,2] Common traditional approaches include simple medial eminence shaving, proximal/distal metatarsal osteotomies, isolated/adjunctive hallux osteotomy, and/or joint fusion(s). Various bone fixation methods can be implemented based on surgeon choice and bunion severity, and these fixation options include cerclage wires, K-wires, bone staples, screws, and/or plating constructs.[3]

Department of Orthopedics, BronxCare Health System, 1650 Grand Concourse, Bronx, NY 10457, USA
E-mail address: dwong@bronxcare.org

Clin Podiatr Med Surg 42 (2025) 103–116
https://doi.org/10.1016/j.cpm.2024.09.002
0891-8422/25/© 2024 Elsevier Inc. All rights are reserved, including those for text and data mining, AI training, and similar technologies.

podiatric.theclinics.com

Table 1
Categorical representation surgical primary bunion procedures

Category	Procedure(s)
Soft tissue	Adductor Release
Exostectomy	McBride

Osteotomy (Metatarsal)	Incisional:
	• Distal
	  ○ Reverdin/Austin
	• Midshaft
	  ○ Scarf
	• Proximal
	  ○ CBWO
	  ○ Cresentric
	Minimally Invasive:
	• Intracapsular
	  ○ First Generation
	    ■ Reverdin-type
	    ■ Unfixated
	• Subcapital
	  ○ Second Generation
	    ■ Transverse
	    ■ Percutaneous K-wire
	  ○ Third Generation
	    ■ Chevron
	    ■ Two screws
	  ○ Fourth Generation
	    ■ Transverse
	    ■ Two screws
	  ○ Fifth Generation
	    ■ Chevron
	    ■ Single screw
	  ○ Sixth Generation
	    ■ Transveron™ osteotomy
	    ■ Single screw (dual-zone)

Joint Destructive	Resection Arthoplasty Joint Replacement Arthrodesis: • First metatarsophalangeal joint • First tarsometatarsal joint (Lapidus)

With the hundred plus surgical bunion treatment options, it's no wonder that recurrence rates are staggering with traditional methods. A 2021 systematic review and meta-analysis by Ezzatvar and colleagues involving 23 studies and 2914 individuals identified 24.86% recurrence rate after open bunionectomy.[4] A 2014 level III consecutive case series of 100 patients who underwent open distal chevron osteotomy observed a 73% radiographic recurrence rate at a mean radiographic follow-up at 7.9 years.[5] Ascertaining the true recurrence rate is likely impossible with the over 150 different bunion surgery methods.[6–8] Nonetheless, the risk for bunion recurrence is acknowledged by both patient and surgeon and the etiology can be diverse or simply unknown.

RECURRENT BUNION CAUSES AND TREATMENTS

It's well accepted that the etiology of recurrence after bunion surgery is multifactorial including specific surgical techniques, bunion severity, patient's foot anatomy/

structure/flexibility, and postoperative compliance.[9] Solving for the many reasons for recurrence can create a dilemma as the revision should not fall into the same prevailing factors that led to the recurrence in the first place. As such, careful history taking and clinical evaluation is important during the work-up and considering the revision plan. It should be mentioned that the recurrent bunion often has secondary resultant issues that impact revision decision making, which include existing scars, adhesions, nerve issues, tendon dysfunction, previous tenotomies, joint contractures, arthrofibrosis, arthrosis, and osseous disfigurement.

Currently, there is no one singular approach to best treat bunion recurrence.[10] Surgical options often involve open incisional osteotomies, joint fusions, first MPJ joint arthroplasty (Keller procedure), and/or first MPJ replacement. Often resultant metatarsal shortening exists from the index operation that might need to be resolved with bone lengthening/grafting. Because of the variable recurrent bunion presentation scenarios causes and multitude of treatment options, as well as the cost of health care delivery, the best treatment has remained unclear.[11]

The Lapidus procedure (first tarsometatarsal joint arthrodesis) has become a widely accepted method for primary bunion repair in the United States and also the go-to method for the recurrent bunion.[12] The ideology of performing Lapidus for revisions is that fusion is nearly recurrence-free but this is just not the case. Moreover, Lapidus procedure comes with a significant recovery phase, which may include a long period of non-weight-bearing use of a cast/boots and crutches for an extended time ranging from several weeks to months. In turn, this can lead to muscle atrophy and prolonged full recovery. Midfoot fusions also have an elevated risk of complications that include scar formation, infection, persistent pain, thrombosis, and limited joint mobility.[13,14]

MODERN MINIMALLY INVASIVE BUNION SURGERY

In recent years, minimally invasive surgery has resurfaced with newer implant technology and techniques making minimally invasive bunion surgery (MIBS) (percutaneous subcapital distal osteotomy with scaffolding screws) a contender for the dominant primary bunion procedure. Several research studies have validated the efficacy and satisfactory outcomes highlighting faster recovery, reduced postoperative pain, small scars (better cosmetics), and preservation of joint motion.[4–6,8,10,15–21] In 2021, Neufeld et al performed an outcome study after MIBS for primary hallux valgus demonstrating radiographic correction (intermetatarsal angle and hallux valgus angle improvement), 5% reoperation rate, and a 94% excellent or good satisfaction rate.[21]

MIBS has seen several iterations (ie, generations) and will likely continue to evolve. The first iteration involved an intracapsular osteotomy of the first metatarsal head with bandage splinting (Isham 1991).[22] The next iteration involved a transverse first metatarsal neck osteotomy with a positional axial percutaneous stabilizing K-wire (Bösch 1990, Giannini 2008).[23,24] The following and most game-changing advancements (ie, third and fourth generations) involved various subcapital osteotomy configurations (chevron or transverse, respectively) of the first metatarsal with internal fixation consisting of 2 percutaneous specialized beveled headed fully threaded bone screws (Redfern and Vernois 2018).[25–28] The most recent evolution (fifth- and sixth generation) that involve a single single screw construct and a stabilizing osteotomy configuration (chevron or Tranveron™) (Blitz 2023). The differentiation between the fifth and sixth generations are based on the osteotomy type and screw type of MIBS screw used. The fifth generation involves either a compressive or non-compressive neutral pitch screw fixation with a chevron osteotomy, whereas the sixth generation involves a specialized (dual-zone) neutral pitch screw fixation with a Transveron™ osteotomy.[29–35]

As surgeons adopt new MIBS and become proficient with primary bunion cases, its use in recurrence bunions will propogate. The logic for this transition into recurrence is rooting in that the satisfactory results with primary bunion surgery would seemingly translate to revision cases. This is no different than how the Lapidus bunionectomy became a standard for primary bunions and then subsequent standard for revisions. New MIBS is becoming the gold standard for its tiny incisions, joint/mobility preservation, minimal insertional hardware (internal to the bone), and ability to immediate weight bearing in a small surgical shoe. Future case reports/studies and research studies on the utility of MIBS in revision are the next logical articles to emerge.

INDICATIONS AND CONTRAINDICATIONS

Modern MIBS is indicated in most recurrent cases where hallux valgus is clinically and radiographically confirmed. The indications include recurrence with or without hypermobility, first MPJ arthritis (so long as there is movement), and previous tarsometatarsal joint (TMTJ) fusion. It seems that MIBS is generally suitable for a large majority of recurrent bunions regardless the index bunionectomy that was performed. It's interestingly also useful for recurrent bunions after MIBS, as the procedure could be repeated.

Like any surgery, there are absolute and relative contraindications. Absolute contraindications may include a medically unfit patient (ie, uncontrolled diabetes with ulcerating neuropathy), vascular impairment (insufficient vascular supply to support healing), mental disorders resulting in instructional noncompliance, uncontrolled infection, and/or others. Relative contradictions include age, bone quality (osteotopenia/osteoporosis), bone stock, non-movement first MPJ arthrosis, neuropathy, and global foot biomechanics. Nonetheless, each patient should be medically evaluated for the suitability of any surgery.

PLANNING AND PREPARATION

Minimally invasive bunion surgery for revision cases involved having the necessary rotary bur, drills, and instrumentation. Also fluoroscopic guidance is a mandatory component, and prefer the use of a smaller unit rather that the large C-arm units. The surgery is generally performed without a tourniquet for the minimally invasive portion, and any preliminary procedure that requires an incision tourniquet can be used.

Frequently, there is surgical hardware of iatrogenic pathology that the surgeon must take into consideration. If the surgeon establishes that completing MIBS osteotomy and screw fixation around the existing hardware is possible, then the hardware can remain in place without extraction. Mixed implant metals should also be considered. If the plates or screws prohibit osteotomy completion or new hardware insertions, then hardware will need to be removed. Depending on the extent and location of the existing hardware, explantation could also be staged. It's preferred to remove the existing hardware by way of percutaneous and small incisions when possible. Some hardware such as plates, embedded stapes/screws will require more traditional standard incisional lengths. It is in the best interest to avoid a situation where the hardware must be removed after an osteotomy has been performed. Hardware removal is challenging enough on a stable osseous structure and can become extremely difficult with an unstable floating metatarsal head (post osteotomy). To avoid being placed into this frustrating predicament, thorough and judicious decision-making during preoperative planning is paramount.

SURGICAL TECHNIQUE

The procedure is carried out under local sedation or general anesthesia in the usual sterile fashion. The entire surgical procedure is performed percutaneously through multiple small (2–5 mm), independent stab incisions. As for tourniquet use, it's again discouraged for the MIBS portion as bleeding acts as a natural coolant for the bur during cutting. An ankle tourniquet may add bulk and interference with the handposition to place the minimally invasive hardware.

Medial Incision and Osteotomy

A small (or percutaneous) medial incision is created over the first metatarsal neck, with necessary hemostatic precautions and care to protect the underlying neurovascular structures. The metatarsal neck is freed of soft tissue attachments using a periosteal elevator. The first metatarsal osteotomy is performed utilizing a Shannon bur under copious irrigation from medial to lateral. The orientation and configuration of the osteotomy is based on surgeon experience and preference. Correction in the sagittal, transverse, and frontal planes are also performed when performing revision MIBS based on the pathology at hand. In some instances, the osteotomy may be oriented to shorten the metatarsal in an effort to improve the range of motion of the first MPJ. However, often revision cases involve a previously shortened first metatarsal and should be considered to not further overly shorten this segment.

Guidewire Placement and Metatarsal Head Translation

A medial second stab incision is made at the first TMTJ. Under fluoroscopic guidance, a guidewire for the anchor screw (4.0 mm primary screw) is placed into the proximal medial portion of the first metatarsal base. It is then driven through the distal lateral cortical portion of the first metatarsal shaft. It is imperative that the wire perforates the lateral cortical wall cortical purchase zone (CPZ) at a safe distance from the metatarsal osteotomy.[32–34] The distal capital fragment is then translated laterally with a translating instrument. With the metatarsal head and sesamoid position corrected and held stable, the guidewire is advanced into the metatarsal head.

Fixation and Bunionectomy

The construct for third & fourth generation involves 2 (dual) first metatarsal screws. One screw stouter (larger diameter, ie, 4.0 mm) is located proximally on the metatarsal and a second smaller (smaller diameter, 3.0 mm) screw is located distal to the first screw. The fifth and sixth generation constructs both involve a single metatarsal screw. The fifth generation involves a single compressive or non-compressive screw with a chevron osteotomy, whereas the sixth generation involves a single dual-zone non-compressive screw with a Transveron™ osteotomy. The decision for surgeons to determine whether or not to perform one or two screw fixation depends on several factors that involve (1) surgeon MIBS experience, (2) bone quality, (3) amount of metatarsal head translation, (4) stability of the construct, (5) placement of the screw(s), and (6) type of screw. A novel innovative screw design developed by Dr. Neal Blitz contains a dual-zone shaft where the screws pitch is intended for the type (density) of bone the screw is engaging.[31] This dual-zone supports a single screw fixation construct.

Surgeons placing a second metatarsal screw might do so through the primary screw incision or an ancillary incision. After the fixation is achieved, the medial translated excess/redundant first metatarsal bone is then shaved and/or resected with the bur of choice. Some surgeons will leave the resected cortical bone as onlay bonegraft.

Lateral Release

The decision to perform a lateral release is purely based on the surgeons experience and clinical presentation after the deformity is reduced. Usually with recurrent bunions, a lateral release is invariably performed. A percutaneous lateral capsular release of the adductor tendon may be performed using a beaver blade or scalpel. One must realize that a lateral release may have already been performed during the initial failed surgery, yielding an anti-climactic soft tissue correction during the revision surgery.

Akin Osteotomy

Percutaneous Akin osteotomy may be added if necessary, again based on surgeon experience and the clinical scenario. Often previous Akin has been performed so it's important to assess the congruency of the hallux interphalangeal joint to the first MPJ. In some cases, the Akin osteotomy may be incomplete and in other situation, a full through-and-through osteotomy to be performed. There are arguments for osteotomy orientation and screw placement, so the surgeon should determine the best configuration based on the presentation.

MINIMALLY INVASIVE BUNION SURGERY CONSIDERATIONS BASED ON INDEX BUNIONECTOMY

The goal of revision bunion surgery is no different than that of a primary bunion. That goal is simple—resolve pain, remove the prominent medial eminence, and straighten the big toe. Recurrent bunions, as mentioned earlier in the article, are often met with preexisting bone deformity (ie, malunion), retained hardware, first MPJ cartilaginous adaption issues/arthrosis, and soft tissue adhesions/constraints. While there are many dozens of primary bunion procedures, the revisions considerations fall/grouped into what index bunion operation was performed. Generally, there are distally based,

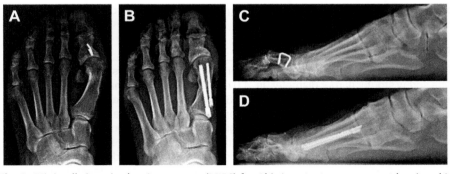

Fig. 1. Minimally invasive bunion surgery (MIBS) for Akin/exostectomy recurrent bunion. (*A, C*) Preoperative radiographs demonstrating bunion recurrence after Akin and exostectomy. Here, the first metatarsophalangeal joint (MPJ) is intact with mild arthritic changes. (*B, D*) Postoperative radiographs after MIBS using 2 metatarsal screw fixation. The deformity is corrected and hallux is rectus. There is robust healing of the MIBS osteotomy (first metatarsal regeneration [FMR] Type III).

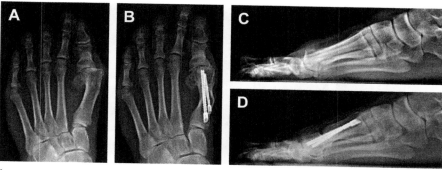

Fig. 2. MIBS for Akin/exostectomy recurrent bunion. (*A, C*) Preoperative radiographs demonstrating bunion recurrence after Akin and exostectomy. The previous Akin was performed without hardware as the osteotomy line is visible. There is moderate radiographic arthrosis of the first MPJ (flattening of the joint) with good supple clinical motion. (*B, D*) Postoperative radiographs after MIBS using 2 metatarsal screw fixation. The hallux is rectus, and the presence of radiographic arthrosis is inconsequential. Note the congruency of the hallux interphalangeal joint and first MPJ due to previous Akin procedure.

proximally based, and Lapidus based recurrences. Each group has a unique set of considerations and challenges that will be discussed.

Considerations for Exostectomy Recurrent Bunions

Simple exostectomy recurrent bunions are the often easiest in this category to treat so long as the functionality of the first MPJ is intact (**Figs. 1** and **2**). In some of these scenarios, the medial eminence resection is often overly aggressive, and the hallux is in a fair amount of abduction. Despite the often staking of the metatarsal head, there is usually good range of motion of the big toe joint. There may or may not be hypermobility of the first TMTJ, but having a pristine midfoot complex makes the MIBS repair more predictable. From an osteotomy standpoint with MIBS, the technique is straightforward. After the fixation is in place, it's important to adequately release/reflect the

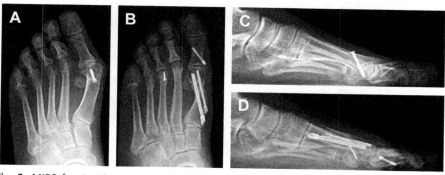

Fig. 3. MIBS for Austin recurrent bunion. (*A, C*) Preoperative radiographs demonstrating bunion recurrence after distal first metatarsal osteotomy with screw fixation. The existing hardware is located centrally within the metatarsal head and would interfere with placement of the MIBS fixation, and therefore would need to be removed. (*B, D*) Postoperative radiographs after MIBS using 2 metatarsal screw fixations and an Akin procedure. The hallux is rectus and recurrent bunion is corrected. There is FMR Type II healing of the first metatarsal.

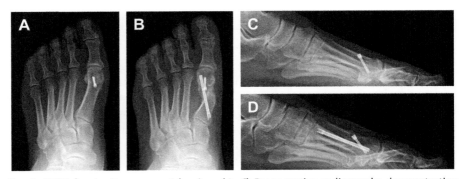

Fig. 4. MIBS for Austin recurrent bunion. (*A, C*) Preoperative radiographs demonstrating bunion recurrence after distal first metatarsal osteotomy with screw fixation. (*B, D*) Postoperative radiographs after MIBS. Here, the existing hardware was left in place requiring the osteotomy to be placed more proximal on the metatarsal and a narrower zone for the MIBS screw to be placed in the metatarsal head. The hallux is rectus and recurrent bunion is corrected.

medial collateral ligament and perform an adductor release given likely long-standing scar tissue of the joint. An akin osteotomy is added as needed.

Considerations for Distally Based Recurrent Bunions

This is the most common revision that is seen in practice because the distal metatarsal osteotomy bunionectomy has been so widespread throughout the last 50 years. Most common presentation is an Austin head procedure (or some variation thereof) with retained hardware (**Figs. 3** and **4**). The head would have been translated 50% on the proximal metatarsal with abductory malunion. The hardware usually involves 1 or 2 dorsal to plantar screws with varying head profiles. Surgical speaking the retained screws can be challenging to remove depending on how embedded the screws head

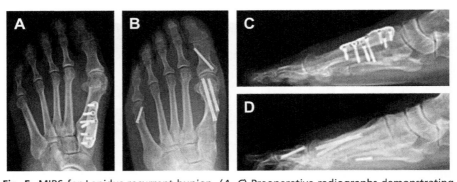

Fig. 5. MIBS for Lapidus recurrent bunion. (*A, C*) Preoperative radiographs demonstrating bunion recurrence after Lapidus with plate fixation. The existing footprint of the hardware requires removal prior to MIBS. Note the first MPJ is without arthrosis, which is often the case after previous Lapidus procedures. (*B, D*) Postoperative radiographs after MIBS using 2 metatarsal screw fixations and an Akin procedure. There is limited ability to translate the head laterally due to the rigidity of the midfoot. The MIBS hardware was placed more distally than typical for this reason. The end result is a healed metatarsal (FMR Type II) and absent bunion.

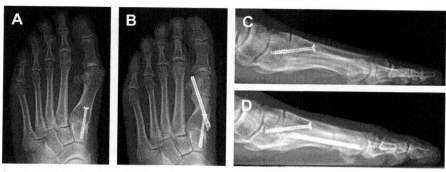

Fig. 6. MIBS for Lapidus recurrent bunion. (*A, C*) Preoperative radiographs demonstrating bunion recurrence after Lapidus with a single screw (dual-zone) fixation. The existing footprint of the hardware is minimal and deeply embedded and would not impede placement of new MIBS fixation. (*B, D*) Postoperative radiographs after MIBS using a single dual-zone metatarsal screw fixation. A stable pseudoarthrosis is present and the metatarsal head is realigned.

in withing the bone, and therefore consideration on leaving the hardware untouched should considered. The existing screw position can affect the location and position of the osteotomy necessitating a more proximal subcapital osteotomy. Hardware that is medially positioned in the metatarsal head will less likely require explantation as it will unlikely interfere with the placement of the new MIBS screw(s). It is possible that the existing hardware could interfere with a second MIBS screw placement; therefore, a single metatarsal screw construct (fifth or sixth generation MIBS) is preferred. Novices at MIBS should strongly consider removing hardware as they may not be proficient at judging metatarsal head shifts with MIBS and could find themselves in a situation where the existing hardware impeding new hardware placement. As stated earlier, it's easiest to remove fixation prior to osteotomy.

Considerations for Proximally/Lapidus Based Recurrent Bunions

The recurrent Lapidus is much more common than most would like to admit, considering that fusion of the first TMTJ is theoretically "curable" for bunions. While fusion quells hypermobility, it does not eliminate it all midfoot motion, and the first metatarsal can deviate medially through the intercuneiform complex if not primarily fused at the index operation. While Lapidus recurrent bunions will require incisional hardware removal as the existing plate(s) and/or screw(s) generally interfere with the MIBS starting point and/or trajectory (**Figs. 5** and **6**). Fortunately, the metatarsal head is often devoid of pre-existing hardware so there is no physical obstacle to work around when docking the MIBS screw(s). Additionally, it is uncommon to deal with overly resected medial eminences associated with Lapidus and the mobility of the big toe joint is often very good.

The most important technical issue when revising Lapidus recurrence is that the first metatarsal position is fixed at the midfoot and there is zero ability to topple the metatarsal base medially. This means the MIBS correction is purely coming from lateralizing the metatarsal head. The nature of MIBS requires that there be "enough" translation between the proximal metatarsal and metatarsal head so that MIBS screw can secure the 2 bones together. Small shift translations make this MIBS construct very difficult to achieve and can easily be the scenario when revising a Lapidus with MIBS. The surgeon should weigh their ability to achieve an adequate

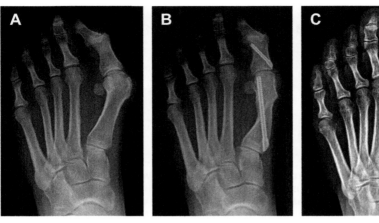

Fig. 7. MIBS for MIBS recurrent bunion. (*A*) Preoperative radiographs demonstrating large bunion deformity, due to a history of trauma. (*B*) Minimally invasive bunion surgery was performed for the index operation and the bunion recurred. There is robust metatarsal healing and room to translate the metatarsal head laterally. (*C*) Repeat MIBS performed using two 4.0 mm screws. Not the realignment and additional translation achieved at 3 months postoperatively. There is Type I FMR healing. (*Image courtesy* of Dr. Neal Blitz.)

translation and may want to consider other revision approaches when this is not possible.

Considerations for Minimally Invasive Bunion Surgery Recurrent Bunions

Despite the low bunion recurrence rate with new MIBS, it is not immune to recurrence (**Fig. 7**). The most common scenario for recurrence is inadequate translation of the capital fragment and/or not fully medializing the proximal metatarsal fragment. While it seems obvious to just perform a Lapidus after an MIBS recurrence, the patient then is subject to all the downsides of the Lapidus (large incisions, bulky palpable plates/screws, joint fusion, and extended period of convalescence). Rather, the MIBS can be repeated allowing for more lateral translation of the metatarsal head and medial toppling of the proximal metatarsal fragment. From a technical standpoint the existing MIBS screw(s) will need to be removed. In many cases, the existing starting point/hole can be used, often a new perforation of CPZ is necessary. Another important consideration when redoing an MIBS with a repeat MIBS is the amount of healing that occurred at the osteotomy site. Those with first metatarsal regeneration (FMR) with healing lateral to the primary screw (FMR Type II & III) will have significant new bone for stabilization of new hardware.[34] In the presence of medial healing (FMR Type I), surgeons need to be more cognizant of new hardware placement to ensure a stable construct.

MINIMALLY INVASIVE BUNION SURGERY POSTOPERATIVE PROTOCOL

There is currently no standard postoperative weight bearing protocol for MIBS, which generally depends on surgeon experience, degree of correction, osteotomy orientation, fixation construct, bone stock, and patient compliance. Most MIBS permits immediate weight bearing in a surgical shoe. With MIBS for revision cases where hardware was explanted (particularly with Lapidus plates and screws), surgeons may prescribe a more restrictive postoperative weight bearing protocol and/or large boots/casts and/or cane/crutches.

MINIMALLY INVASIVE BUNION SURGERY REVISION COMPLICATIONS

There are risks and complications with MIBS just like any other surgical procedure. Failed bunion operations, while uncommon, can happen for a variety of reasons. Understanding these factors is important to limit and manage such consequences.

- *Sub-optimal outcomes:* Inadequate bunion correction is among the risks of MIBS, which include failure to correct the IMA and the HVA of the first MPJ.
- *Fracture(s) aka "Metatarsal Explosion":* Comminuted fractures of the first metatarsal, although rare, can be inevitable despite proper technique. The majority are treated conservatively in an ambulation postoperative surgical shoe based on the identifying fracture classification pattern.[24]
- *Nerve Problems:* There is a possibility of numbness and tingling surrounding any surgical area.
- *Malunion:* The bones may not heal in the desired alignment after surgery. The long-standing soft tissue scarring and cartilaginous joint adaption that can take place over years makes deformity reduction extremely difficult and at times unattainable.
- *Recurrence of the Bunion:* Unfortunately, there is a risk that the bunion may recur again after revision, especially if surgical release of the soft tissues and/or deformity reduction is limited.
- *Hardware Complications:* If screws or pins are used, they may move due to vibration during ambulation and cause discomfort, sometimes necessitating removal. Many times MIBS revisions are performed years after the initial surgery in compromised bones of poor quality. This can create an environment that fosters screw pistoning or even screw pull out while attempting removal.
- *Joint Stiffness:* Despite our best efforts, gross adaptation of the cartilaginous surfaces of the joint may have occurred over time, making stiffness a possibility. There are many causes including pre-existing arthritis, failure to adapt to the newly corrected position of the joint, or postoperative fibrosis and scarring. Although MIBS is less invasive, the joint is still subjected to another traumatic surgical event.
- *Hallux Varus:* There is no way to predict the postoperative forces placed on the first MPJ when revising a previous failed surgery. As opposed to the virgin bunion operation, when a surgeon revises a failed bunionectomy with joint sparing MIBS, hallux varus is a real possibility as one invariably attempts to overcorrect the revision.
- *Infection:* Although it is hypothesized that minimally invasive surgery has lower infection rates due to smaller incisions, there is still a risk of deep infection and osteomyelitis, particularly if bone and/or soft tissue is overheated with the rotary bur.

DISCUSSION

Minimally invasive bunion surgery for recurrent bunions after surgery is a powerful innovative procedure to address the complex unique challenges of these cases. Addressing the recurrent bunion with MIBS provides a more appealing procedure and recovery to an already dissatisfied patient. The surgery involves tiny incisions, immediate weight bearing, and preserves one's joint mobility. While new MIBS is in its infancy for primary bunions, there is a paucity of information for revisions. As such, this paper serves as an important addition to the literature as MIBS becomes more ubiquitous worldwide. Just like MIBS is rapidly becoming the gold standard for primary bunionectomy it will also become the standard for the recurrent bunion.

CLINICS CARE POINTS

- MIBS is a promising surgical technique, demonstrating clinical and radiological outcomes equivalent, if not better than the traditional incisional procedures.
- Most cases of bunion recurrence can be effectively treated with MIBS, regardless of the index bunionectomy performed.
- The functionality of the first MPJ is critical when considering MIBS.
- Soft tissue release at the first MPJ is necessary in most recurrent cases.
- Existing hardware should be considered for explanation on a case-by-case basis, particularly when the existing hardware is located within the metatarsal head.
- Single screw metatarsal fixation (fifth- or sixth generation MIBS) using a stabilizing osteotomy is often preferred with revisions. The fifth generation involves a chevron osteotomy and a compressive or non-compressive screw. The sixth generation involves a Transveron™ osteotomy with a dual-zone screw.
- The postoperative protocol often allows weight bearing in a surgical shoe depending on the extent of previous hardware removal.

ACKNOWLEDGMENTS

Eric Baskin, DPM, Bogdan Grecea, DPM.

DISCLOSURE

Consultant for Voom Medical Devices, Inc.

REFERENCES

1. Hardy RH, Clapham JC. Observations on hallux valgus; based on a controlled series. J Bone Joint Surg Br 1951;33-B(3):376–91.
2. Sanhudo JAV, Pereira TAP. Current trends in fixation techniques. Foot Ankle Clin 2020;25(1):97–108.
3. Clemente P, Mariscal G, Barrios C. Distal chevron osteotomy versus different operative procedures for hallux valgus correction: a meta-analysis. J Orthop Surg Res 2022;17(1):80.
4. Ezzatvar Y, López-Bueno L, Fuentes-Aparicio L, et al. Prevalence and predisposing factors for recurrence after hallux valgus surgery: a systematic review and meta-analysis. J Clin Med 2021;10(24):5753.
5. Pentikäinen I, Ojala R, Ohtonen P, et al. Preoperative radiological factors correlated to long-term recurrence of hallux valgus following distal chevron osteotomy. Foot Ankle Int 2014;35(12):1262–7.
6. Siddiqui NA, LaPorta GA. Minimally invasive bunion correction. Clin Podiatr Med Surg 2018;35(4):387–402.
7. Smyth NA, Aiyer AA. Introduction: why are there so many different surgeries for hallux valgus? Foot Ankle Clin 2018;23(2):171–82.
8. Nair A, Bence M, Saleem J, et al. A systematic review of open and minimally invasive surgery for treating recurrent hallux valgus. Surg J (N Y) 2022;8(4):e350–6.
9. Goh GS, Tay AYW, Thever Y, et al. Effect of age on clinical and radiological outcomes of hallux valgus surgery. Foot Ankle Int 2021;42(6):798–804.

10. Malagelada F, Sahirad C, Dalmau-Pastor M, et al. Minimally invasive surgery for hallux valgus: a systematic review of current surgical techniques. Int Orthop 2019;43(3):625–37.
11. Molloy A, Heyes G. Cost-effectiveness of surgical techniques in hallux valgus. Foot Ankle Clin 2020;25(1):19–29.
12. Ellington JK, Myerson MS, Coetzee JC, et al. The use of the Lapidus procedure for recurrent hallux valgus. Foot Ankle Int 2011;32:674–80.
13. Coetzee JC, Resig SG, Kuskowski M, et al. The Lapidus procedure as salvage after failed surgical treatment of hallux valgus: a prospective cohort study. J Bone Joint Surg Am 2003;85(1):60–5.
14. Grimes JS, Coughlin MJ. First metatarsophalangeal joint arthrodesis as a treatment for failed hallux valgus surgery. Foot Ankle Int 2006;27(11):887–93.
15. de Carvalho KAM, Baptista AD, de Cesar Netto C, et al. Minimally Invasive Chevron-Akin for correction of moderate and severe hallux valgus deformities: clinical and radiologic outcomes with a minimum 2-year follow-up. Foot Ankle Int 2022;43(10):1317–30.
16. Singh MS, Khurana A, Kapoor D, et al. Minimally invasive vs open distal metatarsal osteotomy for hallux valgus - a systematic review and meta-analysis. J Clin Orthop Trauma 2020;11:348–56.
17. Magnan B, Negri S, Maluta T, et al. Minimally invasive distal first metatarsal osteotomy can be an option for recurrent hallux valgus. Foot Ankle Surg 2019; 25(3):332–9.
18. Baskin ES, Luong K, Aamir A, et al. Identification of portals and evaluation of their safeness for MIS arthrodesis of the 1st tarsometatarsal joint. Foot Ankle Surg: Techn, Rep Cases 2023;3(1):100299.
19. Alimy AR, Polzer H, Ocokoljic A, et al. Does minimally invasive surgery provide better clinical or radiographic outcomes than open surgery in the treatment of hallux valgus deformity? A systematic review and meta-analysis. Clin Orthop Relat Res 2023;481(6):1143–55.
20. Ji L, Wang K, Ding S, et al. Minimally Invasive vs. Open surgery for hallux valgus: a meta-analysis. Front Surg 2022;9:843410.
21. Neufeld SK, Dean D, Hussaini S. Outcomes and surgical strategies of minimally invasive chevron/akin procedures. Foot Ankle Int 2021;42(6):676–88.
22. Isham SA. The Reverdin-Isham procedure for the correction of hallux abducto valgus. A distal metatarsal osteotomy procedure. Clin Podiatr Med Surg 1991; 8(1):81–94.
23. Bösch P, Wanke S, Legenstein R. Hallux valgus correction by the method of Bösch: a new technique with a seven-to-ten-year follow-up. Foot Ankle Clin 2000;5(3):485–98, v-vi.
24. Giannini S, Faldini C, Vannini F, et al. The minimally invasive osteotomy "S.E.R.I." (simple, effective, rapid, inexpensive) for correction of bunionette deformity. Foot Ankle Int 2008;29(3):282–6.
25. Vernois J, Redfern D. Percutaneous Chevron; the union of classic stable fixed approach and percutaneous technique. Fuß Sprunggelenk 2013;11:70–5.
26. Redfern D, Vernois J, Legré BP. Percutaneous surgery of the forefoot. Clin Podiatr Med Surg 2015;32(3):291–332.
27. Ferreira GF, Nunes GA, Dorado DS, et al. Correction of first metatarsal pronation in metaphyseal extra-articular transverse osteotomy for hallux valgus correction. Foot & Ankle Orthopaedics 2023;8(3). https://doi.org/10.1177/24730114231198527.
28. Lewis TL, Lau B, Alkhalfan Y, et al. Fourth-generation minimally invasive hallux valgus surgery with metaphyseal extra-articular transverse and akin osteotomy

(META): 12 Month clinical and radiologic results. Foot Ankle Int 2023;44(3): 178–91.

29. Blitz NM. New minimally invasive bunion surgery: easier said than done. Foot Ankle Surg: techn. Rep Cases 2023;3(4):2023–100288.

30. Blitz NM. Game-changing new modern minimally invasive surgery. Foot Ankle Q 2020;31:181–91.

31. Voom Medical Devices, Co. Revcon minimally invasive screw system surgical technique. Available at: https://www.voommedicaldevices.com/files/2023_Voom_OpTech_Complete_Digital_01.pdf.

32. Blitz NM, Grecea B, Wong DT, et al. Defining the cortical purchase zone in new minimally invasive bunion surgery. A retrospective study of 638 cases. J Min Invasive Bunion Surg 2024;1:92777. https://doi.org/10.62485/001c.92777.

33. Blitz NM, Wong DT, Baskin ES. Patterns of metatarsal explosion after new modern minimally invasive bunion surgery. A retrospective review and case series of 16 feet. J Min Invasive Bunion Surg 2024;1:92774. https://doi.org/10.62485/001c.92774.

34. Blitz NM, Wong DT, Grecea B, et al. Characterization of first metatarsal regeneration after a new modern minimally invasive bunion surgery. A retrospective radiographic review of 172 cases. J Min Invasive Bunion Surg 2024;1:92756. https://doi.org/10.62485/001c.92756.

35. Blitz NM. New Minimally Invasive Bunion Surgery: The End-all Be-all Bunion Repair? Clin Podiatr Med Surg 2025;42(1):10–31.

The Unfamiliar Complications of Minimally Invasive Foot Surgery

Kris A. Di Nucci, DPM

KEYWORDS

- Complications • Minimally invasive surgery • Minimally invasive bunion surgery

KEY POINTS

- The likelihood of complications in minimally invasive foot and ankle surgery generally diminishes as a surgeon's proficiency and experience with the procedure(s) increase.
- The evolution of minimally invasive surgery for foot and ankle has transitioned from fixation-free methods to those with limited fixation, advancing to techniques that use specific fixation strategies.
- The risk of malfunction increases for specialized surgical instruments and power tools when excessively stressed, especially by surgeons with less experience.
- Utilizing specific tools, like low-speed/high-torque burrs, avoiding tourniquet hemostasis, and specialized irrigation systems can enhance bone-cutting efficiency and reduce the risk of thermal damage.
- Recognizing a learning curve in minimally invasive surgeries exists, it is not typically associated with negative patient outcomes, but rather with prolonged operating times and a higher dependence on intraoperative radiography.

INTRODUCTION

Minimally Invasive surgery (MIS) has emerged as a transformative approach in the realm of foot and ankle procedures, offering a blend of innovative techniques and minimally invasive interventions. This surgical approach, characterized by smaller incisions and less tissue disruption compared to traditional open surgery, aims to minimize postoperative pain, reduce recovery time, and decrease the risk of infection. However, while MIS presents significant advantages, it is not without its unique set of complications. These complications range from nerve damage to severe metatarsal fractures necessitating a detailed exploration to understand their implications fully. This article delves into the complexities and challenges associated with MIS in foot and ankle surgeries, aiming to provide a comprehensive understanding of its potential

Private Practice, Foot & Ankle Center of Arizona, 7304 E Deer Valley Road #100, Scottsdale, AZ 85255, USA
E-mail address: kadelta24@gmail.com

Clin Podiatr Med Surg 42 (2025) 117–138
https://doi.org/10.1016/j.cpm.2024.09.003
0891-8422/25/© 2024 Elsevier Inc. All rights are reserved, including those for text and data mining, AI training, and similar technologies.
podiatric.theclinics.com

risks and complications. The focus is not only on identifying these issues but also on understanding their underlying causes and the impact they have on patient outcomes, thereby offering valuable insights for both surgeons and patients considering these advanced surgical techniques.

The continuous evolution of surgical technologies and the introduction of new surgical approaches require a phase of adaptation for surgeons to attain proficiency in these techniques. There exists a learning curve that must be surmounted to achieve consistent and dependable outcomes from these surgeries. The capability of a surgeon to minimize complications is closely linked to their adept utilization of educational resources and tools. This approach is essential for enhancing patient outcomes and reducing the risks inherent in the surgical procedure.

The utilization of minimally invasive techniques by foot and ankle surgeons has markedly increased, particularly for correcting bone deformities such as hallux valgus. The MIS management of hallux valgus comparative research and systematic analyses indicates that the clinical results are similar to those of conventional open methods, but with the advantages of lower pain levels, smaller incisions, and possibly faster recovery times.[1–5]

It is essential for surgeons to undergo a comprehensive training process to proficiently execute these methods, which helps in avoiding complications and achieving results that either match or surpass those of traditional open surgeries.[6] Various studies, including those by Lewis TL and Bauman AN, have underscored this point, highlighting that surgeons with greater experience tend to have fewer complications. Baumann's research indicated that an average of 35.5 surgeries, within a range of 27 to 40, is required to achieve competency in MIS for hallux valgus.[7,8] The initial learning phase is often characterized by increased operation time and fluoroscopy usage, but this phase does not necessarily correlate with lower success rates or a higher incidence of complications. This article explores both the common and rare complications that may occur in minimal incision foot surgeries. Given the limited practice of minimal incision surgery, the complications associated with it may be unfamiliar to surgeons who have limited experience in this field.

GENERAL COMPLICATIONS OF FOOT AND ANKLE MINIMALLY INVASIVE SURGERY

In the landscape of foot and ankle MIS, a range of customary and unique complications are encountered, reflecting the intricacies of this surgical approach. Most large cohort outcome studies report complications such as postoperative infections, nerve damage or irritation, and wound dehiscence at a much lower incidence to comparable open surgeries.[9] MIS aims to reduce tissue trauma, decrease the incidence of postsurgical wounds by smaller incisions, retain vascularity of surgical structures by less tissue stripping, and decrease the recovery time to the patient. The presentation and discussion of complications underscore the importance of meticulous surgical technique, comprehensive preoperative planning, and thorough patient assessment to minimize risks and enhance recovery outcomes in foot and ankle MIS.

PATIENT-RELATED FACTORS AND COMPLICATIONS

Patient-related factors play a pivotal role in the risk and manifestation of complications in foot and ankle MIS. Factors such as age, overall health, and the presence of comorbidities such as diabetes mellitus and peripheral vascular disease significantly influence the patient's response to the surgery and the healing process (**Table 1**). Older patients or those with compromised immune systems may experience slower healing and a heightened risk of postoperative infections. Additionally, lifestyle factors,

Table 1
Host factors contributing to minimally invasive surgery complications

Category	Details
Systemic Illnesses	Diabetes
	Chronic steroid use
	Collagen tissue disorder
	Thyroid disorder
	Bone metabolism abnormalities
Skin Health	Peripheral circulation abnormality
Social Habits	Tobacco use
	Alcoholism

including smoking or obesity, can impair wound healing and increase the likelihood of complications. Bone density and quality, often impacted by conditions like osteoporosis, are crucial in surgeries involving bone manipulation, as they can affect the stability of surgical corrections and the risk of fractures. Preexisting foot deformities or previous foot surgeries can also complicate the surgical procedure and recovery. Understanding these individual patient factors is essential for tailoring the surgical approach, anticipating potential complications, and implementing appropriate preventive measures, thereby ensuring a safer surgical experience and optimal recovery for each patient undergoing MIS. In a case series of 16 feet, Blitz and colleagues[10] found "metatarsal explosion" after MIS hallux valgus repair occurred more frequently with thyroid disorders, osteopenia, and increased body mass index.

Skin healing complications can be categorized into host and surgical factors. Preoperative assessment of host factors, which are vital, should occur well in advance of surgery. This includes evaluating the health of the tissue, which is paramount for effective skin healing. Systemic conditions like peripheral arterial disease, diabetes mellitus, peripheral neuropathy, and chronic tobacco use are common contributors to complications in all surgical types.[6,7] Additionally, poor skin quality, such as thin dermal layers from prolonged steroid use or scarring from previous trauma, connective tissue disorders or previous surgeries, can impede healing. These preexisting patient conditions are crucial in determining surgical success and require comprehensive evaluation and management (**Fig. 1**).

Wound complications in surgery are closely tied to a surgeon's skill level and experience. Several factors contribute to surgical proficiency, particularly in MIS. These include patient positioning, muscle memory, and dexterity in using MIS instruments under fluoroscopic guidance, which are essential for accessing the surgical field. Inexperienced surgeons have been shown to require significantly more time for initial surgeries, which can lead to increased wound trauma due to prolonged exposure.[7,8] Moreover, repetitive instrument manipulation in small incisions can cause microtrauma, leading to inflammation, potential bacterial introduction, and increased risk of wound dehiscence or infection. Newcomers to specific MIS techniques may also face challenges related to tissue health, mechanical stress, and thermal injury, which are particularly pertinent in minimal incision surgeries (**Table 2**). These multifaceted reasons for skin healing complications can greatly affect the healing process and the overall success of the surgery.

Wound healing complications in surgery, particularly those attributed to mechanical stress from surgical equipment like drills, can significantly affect the healing process. This stress, arising from both the thermal heat generated during procedures such as over drilling a guidewire and the mechanical irritation caused by the equipment's

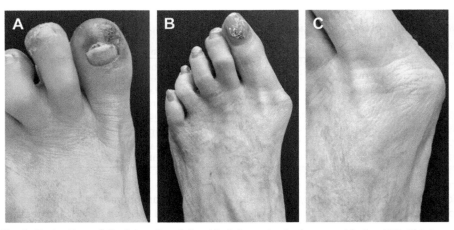

Fig. 1. Evaluation of the integrity of the skin is important when considering MIS. This is an example of a patient with a wound on her great toe from Raynaud's syndrome (*A*). Care must be taken to properly evaluate arterial flow to the surgical site (*B*). In patients with bunion deformities, a close evaluation of the skin and venous system (superficial varicosities and telangiectasia) may reveal fragile skin that should be carefully protected to lessen postoperative wound-healing problems (*C*).

Table 2
Surgery factors contributing to complications in minimally invasive surgery surgery

Factor	Details
Mechanical Stress	Mechanical stress due to thermal heat or mechanical irritation of epidermal tissue, often caused by surgical instruments like drills. Inexperienced surgeons may inadvertently cause skin trauma while focusing on fluoroscopic imaging.
Iatrogenic Injuries	Unintentional abrasions and injuries to the skin during surgery. Too small of incision and increased tension at margins with instrumentation.
Drill Design	Low-profile drills are beneficial for maneuvering around bone prominences. The width and design of the drill can significantly impact wound healing.
Thermal Burns	Lack of burr control and prolonged usage are linked to increased risk of thermal necrosis.
Bur System Innovations	New burr systems include irrigation features to cool the burr, reducing the risk of thermal injury.
Tourniquet Hemostasis	Surgeries, without tourniquet hemostasis, utilize bone bleeding as a method to cool the temperature of the burr. Postoperative surgical hemostasis must be present.
Shannon Bur Design	The Shannon bur is a high-torque, low-speed burr, aimed at minimizing soft tissue injury, including nerve damage. Its design helps to lower the temperature during use, thereby reducing the chance of bone necrosis.

This table outlines various factors that contribute to wound healing complications during surgery, emphasizing the importance of surgeon experience, instrument design, and innovative techniques to minimize these risks.

proximity to sensitive tissue, can lead to thermal injury, cell death, and mechanical abrasions. These factors not only complicate the healing of surgical wounds by introducing additional sites that need to heal but also increase the risk of infection and delay overall recovery. Preventive measures include careful surgical planning, employing techniques that minimize tissue damage, using cooling methods to reduce thermal injury, and ensuring the equipment does not come in close contact with vulnerable tissues to avoid abrasions (**Fig. 2**).

POSTOPERATIVE WOUNDS AND INFECTIONS

Postoperative infections pose a significant risk in all surgical procedures, influenced by a variety of surgical factors. These include the surgeon's technique, the handling of tissues, the duration of the operation, and numerous patient-specific variables. In 1088 MIS hallux valgus surgeries from 17 studies that reported a very high satisfaction rate, Gonzalez and colleagues reported an infection rate of 1.1%.[11–14]

Many different studies have described a lower incidence of postoperative surgical-site infection with MIS surgeries as compared to open surgeries. The studies

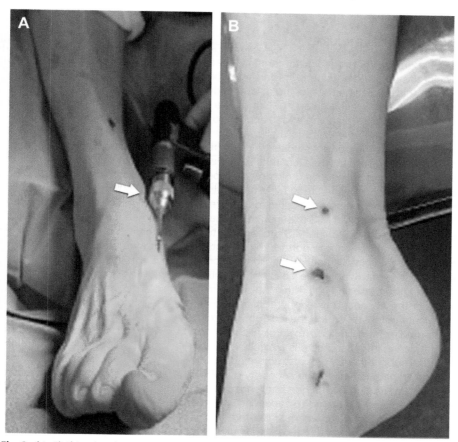

Fig. 2. (*A, B*) Skin abrasions/wounds are an iatrogenic complication caused by the drill being in close proximity to the bony prominences during an MIS bunion repair. Arrows depict the contact points.

conducted by Biz and colleagues,[15] Carranza-Bencano and colleagues,[12] and have demonstrated the effectiveness of minimal incision intramedullary nails for tibiotalo-calcaneal arthrodesis. No cases of wound dehiscence or superficial infection were recorded. One patient had a persistent deep infection with concomitant Charcot neuroarthropathy. Vernois and Refern[16] reported the use of MIS techniques for Lapidus arthrodesis, leading to no postoperative infections and high levels of patient satisfaction. Furthermore, Seat and colleagues[17] meta-analysis on open reduction internal fixation of calcaneal fractures that compared the lateral extensile approach to the minimal incision approach analyzed a total of 2274 fractures across 17 randomized controlled trials. They found that 26 out of 1053 patients (2.47%) treated with minimally incision approach experienced wound complications, significantly lower than 177 out of 1070 patients (16.54%) in the open incision group, marking a significant difference ($P<.001$). Additionally, infection rates were significantly lower in the minimal incision group, with 17 out of 804 patients (2.11%) compared to 47 out of 719 patients (6.54%) in the open incision group, further underscoring the statistical significance ($P<.001$). A retrospective study of hindfoot arthrodeses by Tejero S and colleagues[18] utilized MIS for stage III adult-acquired flatfoot deformity involving 67 feet and revealed no cases of superficial infection or wound dehiscence.

PERIPHERAL NERVE INJURIES

It is imperative for surgeons to carefully release both the subcutaneous and deep fascial tissues before using burrs for osteotomies for removing osteophytes. Overlooking this crucial step raises the risk of inadvertently damaging nerves, which may adhere to the surgical area and be cut by the burrs, underscoring the importance of meticulous surgical planning and execution to avoid/limit nerve injuries.

Cadaveric studies on MIS for hallux valgus reveal varying potential for peripheral nerve injury. Two important studies on nerve injuries demonstrated distinctly different and contrasting results when it comes to nerve injury after MIS hallux valgus repair. In 2016, Yanez and colleagues[19] observed no peripheral nerve damage in a cadaveric study. In 2021 cadaveric study by McGann and colleagues[20], they identified a 50% incidence rate of dorsomedial cutaneous nerve damage that can be directly attributed to the surgeon's limited MIS experience. These findings underscore the importance of experience and precision in MIS procedures to mitigate the risk of nerve injuries.

Cadaveric studies are important to understand the structures are risk during surgery. They are valuable as they highlight the critical role of a trained and experienced surgeon in performing these "blind" procedures. However, it is also important to contextualize these findings within the scope of nonliving (not in vivo) surgery. Factors such as the absence of peripheral circulation, active bleeding in surgeries without tourniquet hemostasis, and the lack of tissue pliability in cadaveric limbs differentiate these studies from live (in vivo) surgical conditions. In vivo surgeries, when using burrs with attached irrigation, there is typically a greater elevation of tissues and separation from the subcutaneous nerve structures than what is observed in cadaveric surgery. This difference underlines the necessity of applying these study findings with caution and acknowledging the unique challenges and conditions present in actual surgical environments as compared to cadaveric specimens.

In an MIS hallux valgus series, Redfern and Vernois[21] reported that 2.4% of patients had some form of nerve-related injury and reported less than 3% dorsomedial cutaneous nerve injury that compares to a reported 3% (Barg and colleagues[22]) with open hallux valgus surgery. In an interesting and important cadaveric study by Dalmau-Pastor and colleagues[23] in 2017, they introduced the innovative "clock method" for pinpointing the locations of the dorsomedial and dorsolateral nerves with MIS hallux valgus surgery. This technique demonstrated that the dorsomedial nerve consistently occupies the area between 12 and 2 o'clock on the right foot, and between 10 and 12 o'clock on the left foot. Conversely, the dorsolateral nerve is reliably located between 12 and 2 o'clock on the left foot, and between 10 and 12 o'clock on the right foot. These findings offer critical insights into the precise anatomic locations of these nerves, providing surgeons with a practical guide to minimize the risk of nerve damage during first-ray surgeries.

PSEUDOBUNION

A "pseudobunion," termed by Blitz and Grecea, is the prominent bulging redundant medial bone that from proximal to the bunion region after minimally invasive bunion surgery (MIBS). The pseudobunion is not a complication perse but iatrogenic unintentional symptomatic prominence that forms as a result of the translatory nature of a new MIBS and of exaggerated by improper resection of the medial ledge of bone. Patients often perceive a pseudobunion as failed surgery as the primary bunion bump was traded for a new extremely symptomatic adjacent symptomatic bony bump. The treatment of pseudobunion generally involves an additional surgery to resect the prominent bone and removal of offending distally based hardware.

To mitigate the risk of a pseudobunion, it is crucial to pay meticulous attention to the placement of the surgical hardware. Ideally, positioning the hardware more proximally than the midline bisection of the first metatarsal to allow for adequate resection of the redundant bone without compromising the hardware present. The following example reveals that a surgical approach involved using a collateral 3.0 mm screw, placed in the redundant area of the metatarsal. Such cases highlight the significance of strategic hardware placement and thorough postoperative evaluation to avoid complications such as the pseudobunion (**Fig. 3**). Using only a single metatarsal screw markedly decreases the risk of a pseudobunion by forgoing the distally based collateral screw that often gives rise to the issue in the first place. The single metatarsal MIBS screw fixation construct has been pioneered by Dr. Neal Blitz and commercialized this method along with innovative dual-zone screw technology where the screws pitch matches the intended bone density.[24,25]

HALLUX VARUS

Hallux varus, a complication arising from MIBS, is uncommon. New MIBS involves lateral translation of the metatarsal head (at times surpassing 100% of the width of the metatarsal) that commonly can realign the hallux to a neutral position making a negative intermetatarsal angle uncommon. Combining a lateral soft tissue release at the first metatarsophalangeal joint with an Akin osteotomy may lead to an overcorrection of the deformity and varus alignment of the hallux. This overcorrection underscores the need for careful surgical planning and execution to balance correction and avoid this complication. In a 2023 systematic review of 1078 cases of MIBS by Gonzalez and colleagues[14], only a single case of hallux varus was identified.

When correcting a hallux valgus deformity, precise assessment of the degree of correction at each stage of the surgery is essential. Performing a lateral release of the first metatarsophalangeal joint, in the authors experience, is to target a slightly abducted toe alignment rather than aiming for a perfectly straight toe. Adopting this approach can play a crucial role in preventing overcorrection, which is a key aspect to consider in ensuring the success and effectiveness of the surgical procedure.

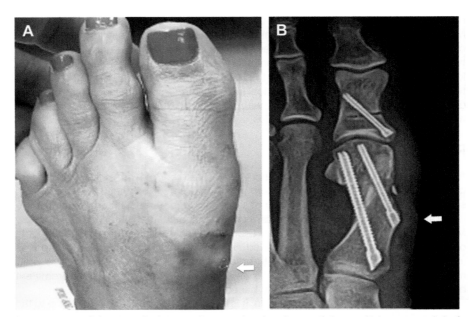

Fig. 3. A "pseudobunion" is the prominent redundant bone of the medial metatarsal shaft that remains after a MIBS correction, which can be symptomatic. (*A*) Clinical image highlighting the location of the pseudobunion (*arrow*). (*B*) Radiographs reveal the underlying prominence (*arrow*).

The postsurgical bandaging may also contribute to hallux varus. Bandaging the toe in an overcorrected or varus position can lead to a less-than-ideal postsurgical alignment. This fact underscores the importance of meticulous surgical planning and technique, coupled with diligent postoperative care. Such comprehensive attention to detail is vital to ensure the most favorable outcomes in the MIS repair of hallux valgus.

DELAYED UNION/NONUNION

Symptomatic delayed/nonunion of the first metatarsal is indeed a concern but is uncommonly seen in hallux valgus MIS procedures. Nonunion has been reported to be exceptionally low at 0.1% to 0.2% of patients.[16] Several factors contribute to the lack of bone healing in such cases:

1. *Inappropriate/excessive use of the burr*: This can lead to thermal necrosis, where the excessive heat generated by the burr damages the bone tissue, impeding its ability to heal. This is the case for osteotomy and/or joint fusions.
2. *Instability of the surgical hardware construct*: If the hardware used to stabilize the bone is not properly secured or is placed in a poor alignment, it can lead to instability, which is detrimental to the healing process.
3. *Pistoning of the metatarsal onto the hardware*: This refers to the movement of the metatarsal bone along the hardware, like a piston, which can disrupt the healing process and prevent the bone from properly uniting. This can occur in 2 particular scenarios, and more likely with osteopenia and/or overactivity. In one scenario, when the proximal hardware is not anchored appropriately in the Cancellous Purchase Zone (CPZ) and is placed into the medullary canal of the first metatarsal.[24] In the other scenario, when the anchor fixation is well seated in the CPZ but the

integrity of the patients bone is unable to withstand the loads and can lead to pistoning of the capital fragment on the screw.

In a recent retrospective radiographic study of 172 feet after MIBS in the *Journal of Minimally Invasive Bunion Surgery* characterized and classified the lateral bony healing (termed First Metatarsal Regeneration [FMR]) with MIBS into 3 types (**Fig. 4**)[26]:

FMR Type I: Involves bone consolidation medial to anchor screw (the primary screw in the fixation construct) and was present in 17.4% of feet,

FMR Type II: Represents both medial and lateral healing around the screw fixation and was present in 42.4% of feet, and

FMR Type III: Characterized by exuberant robust bone formation throughout and was present in 40.1% of feet.

While the study only looked at radiographically healed feet, understanding these different FMR types of bone healing is crucial for surgeons performing MIBS, as it aids in assessing the healing process and planning postoperative care accordingly. Nonunion is an intial concern for those unfamiliar with MIBS and might be identified as a radiographic possibility after 12 weeks postoperatively. Various factors can

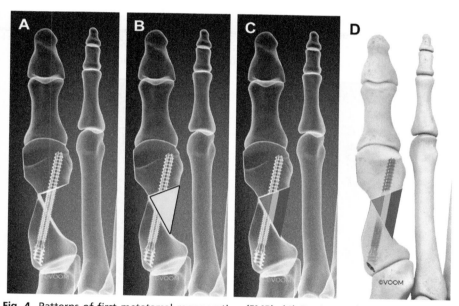

Fig. 4. Patterns of first metatarsal regeneration (FMR). (*A*) Bunion and its correction with minimally invasive bunion surgery (MIBS). (*B*) The realigned capital fragment creates a triangular area, termed the "regeneration triangle" (yellow), lateral to the first metatarsal shaft and proximal to the subcapital osteotomy, where bone regeneration may occur. The regeneration triangle dimensions may vary depending on the size of the bunion and metatarsal head translation in relation to the proximal shaft. (*C, D*) The "anchor screw" (defined as the dominant screw in the fixation construct of a new MIBS that connects the proximal metatarsal segment to the translated metatarsal head) is the reference point that delineates medial versus lateral healing. The 3 regeneration zones are depicted in relation to each other: Type I (red), Type II (blue), and Type III (purple). (*From* Blitz NM, Wong DT, Grecea B, Baskin ES. Characterization Of First Metatarsal Regeneration After New Modern Minimally Invasive Bunion Surgery. A Retrospective Radiographic Review Of 172 Cases. J Min Invasive Bunion Surg. 2024;1:92756. doi:10.62485/001c.92756.)

contribute to this occurrence and are listed in **Table 1**. Premature and excessive stress on the surgical construct is a notable cause, especially in patients with specific conditions such as peripheral neuropathy and compromised bone quality.

Nonunion after MIBS has the similar radiographic hallmark signs of osteotomy/facture/fusion luceny/visibility, absent callus, hypertophic bone, sclerosis, and possibly broken hardware (**Figs. 5** and **6**). It is important to note that the presence of a nonunion does not automatically necessitate revisional surgery. In many cases, delayed consolidation of the bone may still occur over several months. A fibrous asymptomatic nonunion is a satisfactory result. Management strategies in such scenarios may include the use of external bone stimulation devices, offloading the foot to reduce stress on the affected area and the continued use of protective footwear like a fracture shoe or boot. These approaches aim to support the healing process while minimizing the need for additional surgical interventions.

MALUNION

Malalignment in first metatarsal head can indeed be influenced by several factors, including malrotation, elevation, plantarflexion of the metatarsal, and potential hardware failure. In MIBS, the maintenance of joint mobility of the first tarsometatarsal joint (in other words not fusing the midfoot) can compensate for minor deviations in sagittal plane alignment, which might be less tolerable in more rigid constructs typically created in open surgeries. This characteristic of MIBS underscores its advantage in certain clinical scenarios, particularly where maintaining joint mobility is

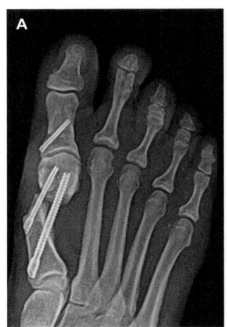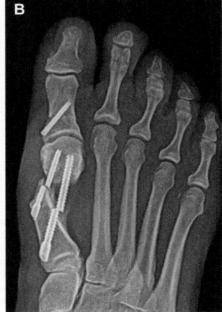

Fig. 5. Radiographic signs of a delayed/nonunion after MIBS. Early postoperative radiographs (A) illustrate some bone callus but incomplete consolidation. Six month radiographs (B) reveal broken hardware confirming the presence of a nonunion. The presence of a radiographic nonunion in the absence of symptoms is often a satisfactory result, so long as the bunion correction remains maintained.

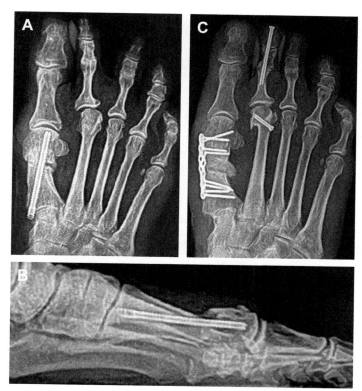

Fig. 6. Elevated malunion identified at 13 weeks after MIBS (*A, B*). The osteotomy site is scle-rotic with compression of the capital fragment resulting in a short first metatarsal. The repair involved autologous bone block distraction at the osteotomy site with plating to restore length. (*C*) Additional second metatarsal shortening osteotomy and hammer toe sur-gery were performed to reestablish the parabola.

beneficial for postoperative function and recovery. In certain cases, the first meta-tarsal may exhibit various positional abnormalities. There are instances, especially when decompression of the first metatarsophalangeal joint is required or preferred to improve its range of motion, where the first metatarsal head might be shortened and plantarflexed.

It is essential to evaluate the sagittal first plane position on the capital fragment early in the postoperative period and after the bone has consolidated. If the malalignment is significant and causing symptoms, revisional surgery may be necessary. An example of this can be seen in **Fig. 7**, which illustrates a case where the first metatarsal is elevated, following an injury where the great toe had a direct injury to the end of the toe resulting in displacement of the head of the metatarsal. This can lead to joint impingement or a dorsal limitation of motion. In such scenarios, revisional surgery was performed to correct the position by reducing the head of the metatarsal to neutral with the placement of additional fixation.

Surgeons must be skilled in distinguishing between a mild elevation, which might be clinically insignificant, and an elevation severe enough to cause impingement and symptomatic issues. Accurate assessment and appropriate surgical intervention are key to ensuring the best possible outcomes for patients with these complex foot

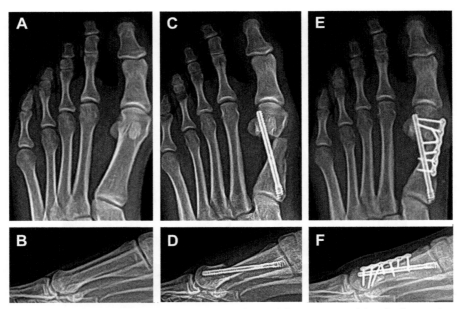

Fig. 7. Radiographic series demonstrating an elevated first metatarsal head after patient injured the foot after MIBS, requiring a revision realignment surgery. Preoperative radiographs (*A, B*) reveal a moderate hallux valgus deformity. Early postoperative radiographs after trauma to the toe result in a dorsal displaced metatarsal head (*C, D*). Untreated may lead to symptomatic malunion resulting impingement of the first metatarsal phalangeal joint and lesser metatarsal overload. Revision radiographs of the open reduction internal fixation of the first metatarsal demonstrate realignment of the displacement while maintaining the initial bunion correction position (*E, F*).

deformities. In surgical procedures of the first metatarsal, the osteotomy technique used can significantly influence the postoperative position of the metatarsal. When a transverse (also known as flat cut) osteotomy that lacks a plantar shelf is performed, there is a tendency for the elevation of the first metatarsal to increase. In these cases, the use of dual screw fixation is considered to provide an additional point of stabilization.

HARDWARE COMPLICATIONS

Vernois and Redfern introduced a stable rigid screw fixation construct (using two minimally invasive chamfered head bone screws(s)) to a subcapital osteotomy, which is the method and construct that sprouted new modern MIBS techniques.[27] Previous large cohort studies have found up to 40% of the total complications of MIS surgery that were hardware related.[28,29] Holme and colleagues[30] reported on a series of 40 patients with consecutive MIBS who had 10 complications postoperatively and 4 were hardware related with Akin screw irritation. The beveled head bone screw designed for MIBS surgery has lowered this particular hardware complication rate. The tapered head design of these screws allows them to be more seamlessly integrated with the natural contour of the metatarsal and phalangeal anatomy, leading to less prominence and potentially reduced irritation.

These factors underscore the need for careful planning and precision in the placement of hardware during MIBS. The benefits of the newer hardware designs and accurate screw placement minimize complications and optimize patient outcomes. Absolutely, these considerations indeed underscore the critical importance of meticulous surgical technique and careful decision-making in MIBS. The surgeon's approach to managing the removal of redundant bone and the strategic placement of hardware is pivotal in preventing complications such as screw loosening, failure, and the development of a pseudobunion.

Surgeons must strike a delicate balance between adequately correcting the deformity and maintaining the structural integrity of the bone and surrounding tissues. This involves not only the technical aspects of the surgery itself but also preoperative planning and postoperative management. Understanding the unique aspects of each patient's anatomy and pathology is crucial for tailoring the surgical approach to their specific needs for an optimal result for the size of the deformity.

RECURRENCE

Recurrence is a common complication after open hallux valgus with a recent meta-analysis finding a recurrence rate as high as 24.9% for open hallux valgus correction.[7] The recurrence rate after MIBS has been reported from 0% to 2.2%, a very low rate when compared to open methods.[14,27,29] Importantly, the number of recurrences that had to be revised in one study was 0.6% (7 out of 1088). In contrast, Barg and colleagues'[22] systematic review of open hallux valgus surgical correction reported a recurrence rate of 4.9%, with the distal metatarsal osteotomies recurrence rate of 4.1%.

A probable reason for the very low recurrence rate with MIBS is due to the locking with first tarsometatarsal joint without arthrodesis[31] (**Fig. 8**). The ability to stabilize the first tarsometatarsal with transverse plane locking is a new concept known to MIBS surgeons

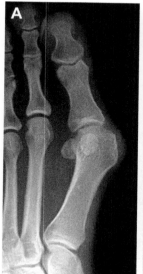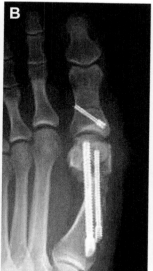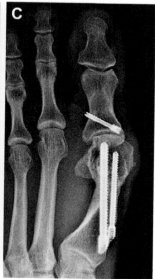

Fig. 8. Bunion recurrence after MIBS due to incomplete locking of the first tarsometatarsal joint. Preoperative radiograph of large bunion deformity (A). Early postoperative radiograph after MIBS with lateralization of the metatarsal head with excellent sesamoid position (B). Recurrent bunion after MIBS with increased intermetatarsal angle, loss of sesamoid position, and abduction of the hallux (C). In this case, the recurrence is attributed to not fully locking the first tarsometatarsal joint at the index operation. (*Image Courtesy* of Dr. Neal Blitz.)

but not commonly ascribed with traditional open hallux valgus surgeons. Translation of the first metatarsal head from 50% to greater than 100% of the width of the metatarsal head seems to lock the hypermobility of the first tarsometatarsal (TMT) Joint.

INSTRUMENT FAILURE

In MIS procedures, particularly in procedures involving bone cutting and manipulation, the instruments employed are subjected to considerable forces. This places high stress on the instruments, which can lead to potential instrument failure/breakage. For example, burs, essential tools in MIS, can break under such conditions, as depicted in **Fig. 9**. Other instruments, like guidewires and drills, are also susceptible to failure when subjected to excessive stress.

The durability of surgical instruments like burrs, guidewires, and drills is not unlimited. Each instrument has a threshold for usage, beyond which the risk of failure increases. Surgeons and surgical teams must be mindful of the recommended guidelines for the usage of these instruments. Exceeding these guidelines can strain the instruments beyond their designed capacity, leading to potential failure.

Surgeons, particularly those who are relatively inexperienced with using low-speed/high-torque burs in surgery, might be inclined to apply excessive torque to the bur during bone cutting. This over leveraging, often done in an attempt to expedite the bone-cutting process, can unfortunately lead to bur breakage. It is crucial for surgeons to understand and respect the limitations of these tools.

To avoid such issues, the following practices are recommended:

1. *Slow and controlled cutting*: The bur should be allowed to cut through the bone in a slow and controlled manner. Rushing the process by applying too much force can be counterproductive, leading to equipment failure.

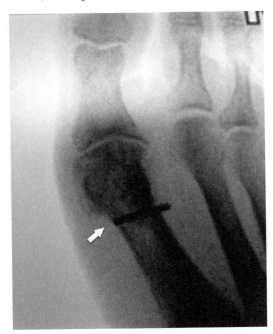

Fig. 9. Broken 2 mm Shannon bur during the performance of the first metatarsal osteotomy in a MIBS correction.

2. *Minimizing heat generation*: Using the bur slowly and steadily helps in limiting the generation of excessive heat. Overheating can cause damage to both the bone (such as thermal necrosis) and the bur.
3. *Ensuring proper cut alignment*: A controlled approach allows for more accurate and precise cuts. Quick, forceful movements can lead to misalignment, affecting the outcome of the surgery.
4. *Understanding tool capabilities*: Surgeons should be familiar with the specifications and recommended usage guidelines for the burs they are using. This includes understanding the optimal speed and torque settings.
5. *Regular instrument check and maintenance*: Regularly checking the condition of the burrs and maintaining them as recommended by the manufacturer can prevent premature wear and breakage.

These practices not only extend the lifespan of the surgical tools but also contribute to a safer surgical environment and better outcomes for patients. It is part of the surgical skill set to understand and adapt to the limitations of the tools being used, ensuring their optimal and safe use in all procedures.

Indeed, in the event that instruments break during surgery, having a plan for retrieval is crucial. Commonly, broken instrument pieces can be retrieved using tools such as hemostats and probes. These tools allow the surgeon to carefully navigate and extract the broken piece without causing additional harm or disruption to the surgical area. For surgeons, being prepared for these eventualities is a critical aspect of surgical planning. This preparation involves

1. *Understanding and anticipating potential complications*: Surgeons should be aware of the types of complications that can arise with the use of various instruments, including the likelihood and consequences of instrument breakage.
2. *Having the right tools on hand*: Ensuring that tools like hemostats and probes are readily available in the operating room can expedite the retrieval process and minimize the interruption to the surgery.
3. *Training and practice*: Surgeons should be trained in and practice the techniques for safely and effectively retrieving broken instrument pieces. This might include training sessions or simulations that mimic such scenarios.
4. *Developing a systematic approach*: Having a standardized approach or protocol for dealing with instrument breakage can help maintain calm and efficiency during these unexpected events.
5. *Effective team communication*: Clear and calm communication with the surgical team is essential during these situations. The team should be aware of the protocol and each member's role in resolving the complication.

Being prepared for instrument breakage and knowing how to handle such situations safely and effectively is essential for ensuring the best possible outcomes for patients. This readiness is part of the broader skill set required for surgeons, particularly those specializing in MIS, where the working environment is often more challenging due to the nature of the procedures and the tools used.

METATARSAL EXPLOSION IN MINIMALLY INVASIVE BUNION SURGERY

A newly described significant postoperative complication during MIBS is a fracture of the first metatarsal that resembles an explosion. This was first described and highlighted in a retrospective review by Blitz and colleagues[10], which identified factors linked to this complication. The study categorized 3 distinct types of "metatarsal explosions," each associated with specific postoperative complications. The study highlighted the importance of the exit of the hardware at the lateral cortex of the first metatarsal and maintaining uninterrupted length of the CPZ. In addition, the use of 2 metatarsal screws carried an increased the risk of a more severe metatarsal explosion ($P<.05$). The types of metatarsal explosions are classified into Types I, II, and III (**Fig. 10**). The distribution among these types was 50% for Type I, 31% for Type II, and 19% for Type III.

In Type I explosions, there is a fracture at the lateral cortex of the first metatarsal at the CPZ. The alignment of the metatarsal and the hardware remain intact and the condition is treated with protecting the metatarsal. There is partial compromise of the hardware, and without malalignment of the surgery, revisional surgery is often not necessary.

In Type II explosions, there is a feature described as the "double metatarsal sign." This is describing a specific fracture alignment where a vertically oriented fracture originates in the mis-first metatarsal shaft and extends to the first tarsometatarsal joint. This fracture has the potential to be unstable and each pattern must be thoroughly evaluated. Type II explosion fractures present unique challenges due to their instability and joint involvement. Therefore, a comprehensive and meticulous approach to surgical management and postoperative care is essential for optimal patient outcomes.

The most severe type of explosion metatarsal fractures are Type III. These fractures are the most severe and can be unstable (**Fig. 11**). The fracture pattern is described as

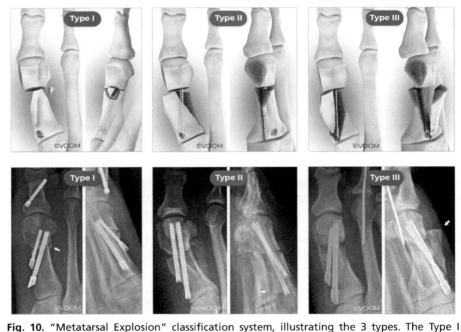

Fig. 10. "Metatarsal Explosion" classification system, illustrating the 3 types. The Type I metatarsal explosion occurs at the screw osteotomy interface of the distal lateral corner of the metatarsal shaft, creating the pathognomonic "fleck" sign. The Type II metatarsal explosion splits the metatarsal shaft in half in the transverse plane (preserving the screws insertion site in the base) but extends into the first tarsometatarsal joint, creating the pathognomonic "double metatarsal sign." The Type III metatarsal explosion also splits the metatarsal in the transverse plane but the fracture line travels along the plane of the screw, creating a "large or butterfly fragment" or "crocodile effect" of the dorsal metatarsal shaft. (*From* Blitz NM, Wong DT, Baskin ES. Patterns of Metatarsal Explosion After New Modern Minimally Invasive Bunion Surgery. A Retrospective Review and Case Series of 16 Feet. J Min Invasive Bunion Surg. 2024;1:92774. doi:10.62485/001c.92774.)

a "butterfly fragment(s)" and occurs along the orientation of the fixation, which creates a large dorsal fragment of the metatarsal shaft. The management of these fractures involves specific and complex surgical intervention due to their instability.

1. *Two plane plate fixation*: Given the significant instability of Type III fractures, they commonly require 2 plane plate fixation. This approach involves using surgical plates to stabilize the fracture in 2 different planes, providing a more robust fixation to accommodate the complexity and instability of the fracture.
2. *Supplementary bone grafting*: Often, these fractures necessitate additional bone grafting. This is particularly important in cases where there are bone deficits resulting from bone excision during the initial procedure or due to the comminution (breaking of the bone into multiple pieces) associated with the fracture. Bone grafting helps in filling these deficits, facilitating proper bone healing and structural integrity.
3. *Careful surgical planning and execution*: The surgical management of Type III fractures requires meticulous planning and precision in execution. The surgeon must consider the best approach for plate fixation and the optimal type and source of bone graft to maintain length of the metatarsal.
4. *Monitoring and managing complications*: Given the severity of these fractures, there is a heightened risk of complications such as nonunion, infection, or hardware failure. Close postoperative monitoring and management are essential.

The concept of maintaining an adequate distance between the osteotomy and the perforation point of the anchor screw (termed cortical runway) within the CPZ is

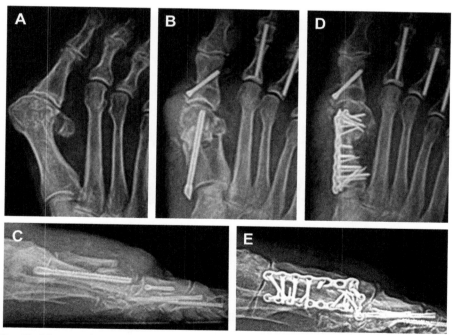

Fig. 11. Metatarsal explosion Type III undergoing open reduction internal fixation (ORIF). Radiograph of preoperative hallux valgus deformity (*A*). Postoperative metatarsal explosion (Type III) with hallmark features of the "double metatarsal sign" on the anteroposterior radiograph (*B*) and the "butterfly fragment" on the lateral radiograph (*C*). Status post-ORIF with 2 plate plating of the first metatarsal (*D, E*).

important when trying to mitigate metatarsal bone complications, such as fractures or "explosions." Based on a retrospective radiographic review study of 638 MIBS cases, Blitz and colleagues[10] mapped our defined "stability regions" within the CPZ (**Fig. 12**) and suggested a cortical runway of 6.6 mm or less would be the "no-go zone" where fixation fractures might be more risky. A cortical runway in the more proximal CPZ stability regions may minimize risk of subsequent fixation failure or metatarsal explosion.

TECHNOLOGICAL ADVANCES AND EQUIPMENT IN MINIMALLY INVASIVE SURGERY

The field of MIS for foot and ankle procedures has witnessed significant technological advances and the development of specialized equipment, which have been instrumental in enhancing surgical precision and patient outcomes. Innovations such as

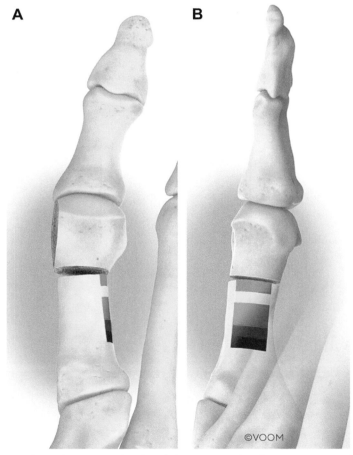

Fig. 12. Cortical purchase zone (CPZ) stability region classification system. The regions closest to the osteotomy carry a higher risk for screw instability, whereas screws furthest from the osteotomy have less risk. Danger region (red), vulnerable region (yellow), standard region (green), safety region (purple), and the security region (blue). Top down (*A*) and medial views (*B*). (*From* Blitz NM, Grecea B, Wong DT, Baskin ES. Defining the Cortical Purchase Zone in New Minimally Invasive Bunion Surgery. A Retrospective Study of 638 Cases. J Min Invasive Bunion Surg. 2024;1:92777. doi:10.62485/001c.92777.)

specialized instruments, like low speed and high torque burrs, have facilitated more efficient bone cutting with reduced risk of thermal necrosis. Additionally, custom-designed screws and fixation devices have been developed to provide better stability and alignment in the foot and ankle. These technological advancements not only aid in reducing the incidence of complications but also contribute to shorter operative times and quicker recovery periods. As these technologies continue to evolve, they promise to further refine MIS techniques, making surgeries more effective and safer for patients.

POSTOPERATIVE MANAGEMENT AND COMPLICATION RESOLUTION

Effective postoperative management is crucial in mitigating complications and ensuring a successful recovery following foot and ankle MIS. Early detection and pro-active management of complications are key. This involves regular monitoring for signs of infection, nerve dysfunction, or improper healing. In cases where complications arise, such as nonunion of bones or postoperative infections, timely intervention is crucial. This may range from administering antibiotics to address infections to potential revisional surgery for more severe complications such as misalignments or hardware failures.

SUMMARY

In conclusion, while MIS in foot and ankle procedures presents a forward-thinking approach with numerous benefits, including reduced recovery times and minimal scarring, it also brings its own set of unique complications. These range from postoperative infections to nerve damage and require careful consideration. The success of MIS in this specialized field hinges not only on the surgeon's expertise and the meticulous application of surgical techniques but also on a thorough understanding of patient-specific factors that may influence outcomes. As MIS continues to evolve, with technological advancements and improved surgical methods, the potential for reducing these complications increases. However, the importance of patient education, diligent postoperative care, and a personalized approach to each case remains paramount. Ultimately, the goal is to balance the innovative advantages of MIS with a deep commitment to patient safety and quality care, ensuring the best possible outcomes for those undergoing foot and ankle surgery.

SUMMARY

Throughout its history, MIS in foot and ankle surgery has evolved from simple beginnings to a highly sophisticated field of medical science. This journey has been marked by a persistent quest to minimize patient trauma and enhance recovery, driven by technological advancements and a deepening understanding of the biomechanics of the foot and ankle. After examining the various complications associated with MIS, it is evident that surgeons with extensive experience and additional training have been successful in minimizing significant complications. The complications discussed in this review reflect current trends published in the literature and align with my personal experiences as a surgeon practicing these techniques. As the adoption of these procedures increases, the authors can anticipate further advancements in equipment, techniques, and implantable hardware. Many proficient surgeons possess the capability to recommend and improve these techniques, with some still at the beginning of their journey in MIS. Like any surgical procedure, the risk of complications is inherent, but with expertise and diligence, these risks can be significantly reduced or even avoided. Surgical skills, much like any other skills, improve with experience. Continual enhancement of our techniques, training, and implants is crucial in the field of MIS surgery. These aspects are integral to refining our practices, ultimately benefiting our patients. The evolution of surgical methods is a testament to the commitment to advancing patient care and outcomes.

CLINICS CARE POINTS

- The learning curve for a new surgeon performing MIS is predictable and competency and improved outcomes are shown with close mentors during the learning process.
- Familiarization of the new surgeons with the surgical instruments, devices, and hand techniques improves the initial adaptation to the procedures and lessens operative time.
- MIS techniques have shown comparable or even superior outcomes to traditional open surgery with similar to less complication rates with MIS surgery.
- Recognition of the current limitations of MIS surgery is important for each surgeon to understand the risks to the patient and potentially leading to poor outcomes.
- Over the next 5 to 10 years with the significant interest in MIS surgery, new techniques, new devices, and equipments will afford patients improved outcomes, less operative time, and quicker recoveries.

DISCLOSURE

K.A. Di Nucci is a consultant for Voom Medical Devices, Inc and Deputy Editor for the *Journal of Minimally Invasive Bunion Surgery*, a publication of Voom Medical Devices, Inc.

REFERENCES

1. Bia A, Guerra-Pinto F, Pereira BS, et al. Percutaneous osteotomies in hallux valgus: a systematic review. J Foot Ankle Surg 2018;57(1):123–30.
2. Maffulli N, Longo UG, Oliva F, et al. Bösch osteotomy and scarf osteotomy for hallux valgus correction. Orthop Clin North Am. 2009;40(4):515–24.
3. Malagelada F, Sahirad C, Dalmau-Pastor M, et al. Minimally invasive surgery for hallux valgus: a systematic review of current surgical techniques. Int Orthop 2019;43(3):625–37.
4. Siddiqui NA, LaPorta G, Walsh AL, et al. Radiographic outcomes of a percutaneous, reproducible distal metatarsal osteotomy for mild and moderate bunions: a multicenter study. J Foot Ankle Surg 2019;58(6):1215–22.
5. Singh MS, Khurana A, Kapoor D, et al. Minimally invasive vs. open distal metatarsal osteotomy for hallux valgus: a systematic review and meta-analysis. J Clin Orthop Trauma 2020;11(3):348–56.
6. Kaufmann G, Dammerer D, Heyenbrock F, et al. Minimally invasive versus open chevron osteotomy for hallux valgus correction: a randomized controlled trial. Int Orthop 2019;43(2):343–50.
7. Lewis TL, Robinson PW, Ray R, et al. The Learning curve of third-generation percutaneous chevron and akin osteotomy (PECA) for hallux valgus. J Foot Ankle Surg 2023;62(1):162–7.
8. Baumann AN, Walley KC, Anastasio AT, et al. Learning curve associated with minimally invasive surgery for hallux valgus: a systematic review. Foot Ankle Surg 2023;27. S1268-7731(23)00152-2.

9. Lu J, Zhao H, Liang X, et al. Comparison of minimally invasive and traditionally open surgeries in correction of hallux valgus: a meta-analysis. J Foot Ankle Surg 2020;59(4):801–6.

10. Blitz NM, Wong DT, Baskin ES, Patterns of Blitz NM, Wong DT, Baskin ES. Patterns of metatarsal explosion after new modern minimally invasive bunion surgery. a retrospective review and case series of 16 feet. J Min Invasive Bunion Surg 2024;1:92774. https://doi.org/10.62485/001c.92774.

11. Coleman MM, Abousayed MM, Thompson JM, et al. Risk factors for complications associated with minimally invasive medial displacement calcaneal osteotomy. Foot Ankle Int 2021;42:121–31.

12. Carranza-Bencano A, Tejero S, Del Castillo-Blanco G, et al. Minimal incision surgery for tibiotalocalcaneal arthrodesis. Foot Ankle Int 2014;35(3):272–84.

13. Reddy SC, Schipper ON, Li J. The effect of chilled vs room temperature irrigation on thermal energy dissipation during minimally invasive calcaneal osteotomy of cadaver specimens. Foot Ankle Orthop 2022;7(4). https://doi.org/10.1177/24730114221136548.

14. Gonzalez T, Encinas R, Johns W, et al. Minimally invasive surgery using a shannon burr for the treatment of hallux valgus deformity: a systematic review. Foot Ankle Orthop 2023;8(1). 24730114221151069.

15. Biz C, Hoxhaj B, Aldegheri R, et al. Minimally invasive surgery for tibiotalocalcaneal arthrodesis using a retrograde intramedullary nail: preliminary results of an innovative modified technique. J Foot Ankle Surg 2016;55(6):1130–8.

16. Vernois J, Redfern D. Lapidus, a percutaneous approach. Foot Ankle Clin 2020; 25:407–12.

17. Seat A, Seat C. Lateral extensile approach versus minimal incision approach for open reduction and internal fixation of displaced intra-articular calcaneal fractures: a meta-analysis. J Foot Ankle Surg 2020;59(2):356–66.

18. Tejero S, Carranza-Pérez-Tinao A, Zambrano-Jiménez MD, et al. Minimally invasive technique for stage III adult-acquired flatfoot deformity: a mid- to long-term retrospective study. Int Orthop 2021;45(1):217–23.

19. Yañez Arauz JM, Del Vecchio JJ, Codesido M, et al. Minimally invasive akin osteotomy and lateral release: anatomical structures at risk-a cadaveric study. Foot 2016;27:32–5.

20. McGann M, Langan TM, Brandão RA, et al. Structures at risk during percutaneous extra-articular chevron osteotomy of the distal first metatarsal. Foot Ankle Spec 2021;14(1):19–24.

21. Redfern D, Vernois J, Legré BP. Percutaneous surgery of the forefoot. Clin Podiatr Med Surg 2015;32(3):291–332.

22. Barg A, Harmer JR, Presson AP, et al. Unfavorable outcomes following surgical treatment of hallux valgus deformity: a systematic literature review. J Bone Joint Surg Am 2018;100(18):1563–73.

23. Dalmau-Pastor M, Vega J, Malagelada F, et al. An anatomical study of nerves at risk during minimally invasive hallux valgus surgery. J Vis Exp 2018;(132):56232.

24. Blitz NM, Grecea B, Wong DT, et al. Defining the cortical purchase zone in new minimally invasive bunion surgery. A retrospective study of 638 cases. J Min Invasive Bunion Surg. 2024;1:92777. https://doi.org/10.62485/001c.92777.

25. Voom Medical Devices, Co. Revcon minimally invasive screw system surgical technique. Available at: https://www.voommedicaldevices.com/files/2023_Voom_OpTech_Complete_Digital_01.pdf.

26. Blitz NM, Wong DT, Grecea B, et al. Characterization of first metatarsal regeneration after a new modern minimally invasive bunion surgery. A retrospective

radiographic review of 172 cases. J Min Invasive Bunion Surg. 2024;1:92756. https://doi.org/10.62485/001c.92756.

27. Vernois J, Redfern D, GRECMIP the. Percutaneous Chevron: the union of classic stable fixed approach and percutaneous technique. Fuß & Sprunggelenk 2013; 11(2):70–5.

28. Ezzatvar Y, pez-Bueno L L, Fuentes-Aparicio L. Due.as L. Prevalence and predisposing factors for recurrence after hallux valgus surgery: a systematic review and metaanalysis. J Clin Med 2021;10(24):5753.

29. Isham SA. The Reverdin-Isham procedure for the correction of hallux abducto valgus. A distal metatarsal osteotomy procedure. Clin Podiatr Med Surg 1991; 8:81–94.

30. Holme TJ, Sivaloganathan SS, Patel B, et al. Third-generation minimally invasive Chevron Akin osteotomy for hallux valgus. Foot Ankle Int 2020;41(1):50–6.

31. Nunes GA, Carvalho K, Ferraz GF, et al. Minimally invasive chevron akin: locking of the metatarsal-cuneiform joint. Foot Ankle Orthop 2022;7(4). 2473011421S00857.

Minimal Incision Management of Rearfoot & Ankle Trauma

Dhavel D. Chauhan, DPM, AACFAS[a], Nehal Modha, DPM, AACFAS[b], Calvin J. Rushing, DPM, FACFAS[c],*

KEYWORDS

- Ankle fracture • Intramedullary fibular nail • Neuropathic fracture
- Intramedullary fixation • Minimally invasive surgery • MIPO
- Tibiotalocalcaneal arthrodesis

KEY POINTS

- Minimally invasive surgery has an important role in rearfoot and ankle trauma treatment by reducing the risk of soft tissue and infectious complications, and providing outcomes equivalent to open approaches.
- Fractures can be reduced and stabilized with advanced techniques and intraoperative fluoroscopic and indication-specific orthopedic hardware.
- Minimally invasive percutaneous osteosynthesis (MIPO) plating and novel intramedullary fibular nailing is an accepted option to stabilize and span fractures using small incisional portals.
- Calcaneal fractures that are treated with minimal invasive methods lessen risk of incisional dehiscence complications seen with the standard lateral extensile approach.
- Primary arthrodesis for charcot neuropathic ankle fractures using a transportal retrograde tibiotalocalcaneal nailing can be considered in this challenging patient population.

INTRODUCTION

Large incisional "traditional" open approaches to orthopedic trauma have been attributed to delayed wound healing, dehiscence, and surgical site infection (SSI).[1–3] The incidence of SSI has been shown to exceed the rates reported for hand surgery, total shoulder arthroplasty, total hip arthroplasty, and total knee arthroplasty.[4–7] These complications increase hospital length of stay, number of re-operations, and readmission rates, adversely impacting both the quality and cost of health care delivery.[8]

Various strategies have been implemented to mitigate complications, including minimally invasive techniques/approaches, preoperative skin antisepsis, practice

[a] Dallas Advanced Foot and Ankle Reconsruction Fellowship, Dallas, TX, USA; [b] McKinney Footcare, 5337 West University Drive Suite 100, Mckinney, TX, USA; [c] Dallas Orthopedic and Shoulder Institute, 222 South Collins Road Suite 101, Sunnyvale, TX 75182, USA
* Corresponding author.
E-mail address: calvin.rushing@mymail.barry.edu

Clin Podiatr Med Surg 42 (2025) 139–152
https://doi.org/10.1016/j.cpm.2024.09.001
0891-8422/25/© 2024 Elsevier Inc. All rights are reserved, including those for text and data mining, AI training, and similar technologies.
podiatric.theclinics.com

improvement strategies, preoperative and postoperative prophylactic antibiotics, surgical checklists, and differing professional society initiatives (ie, Surgical Care Improvement Project, National Surgical Quality Improvement Program, MusculoSkeletal Infection Society and Joint Commission National Patient Safety Goals).[2,3,7–10] Minimally invasive surgery, when compared to open traditional surgery, has demonstrated lower complication rates, less pain, faster recovery, and superior cosmesis.

The focus of this article is to outline the various applications of minimally invasive surgery applications for rearfoot and ankle trauma. The surgical management and decision-making is often guided by severity of the injury and the patient's age, medical comorbidities (ie, diabetes), and importantly the limbs sensory status (ie, peripheral neuropathy). As such, for neuropathic ankle fractures, primary arthrodesis is often favored with a transportal retrograde tibiotalocalcaneal arthrodesis. Ankle fractures in the sensate individual can be managed with a minimal incision approach of minimally invasive percutaneous osteosynthesis (MIPO) and/or intramedullary fibular (IMF) nailing.

INTRAMEDULLARY FIBULAR NAILING

Over the past decade, minimally invasive ankle fracture fixation using IMF nails has continued to gain popularity and acceptance for distal fibular fractures. Often performed as an arthroscopically assisted surgery, this intramedullary minimal incisional approach has been shown to allow for earlier weightbearing (load sharing construct), reduced wound complications (less dissection), better union rates (preservation of the periosteum), and the absence of prominent hardware, compared to traditional plate/screw fixation.[11–17] Moreover, clinical outcomes are equivalent with an overall lower cost of health care delivery, given fewer complications, less reoperations, and lower rates of readmission.[11–13,16]

Various IMF nail devices have been reported in the literature including smooth wires, Steinmann pins, fully threaded cortical screws, locking nails, and fibular specific nails. First generation fibular nailing devices consist of non-fibular specific implants. Second and third generation devices are fibular specific, with the latter incorporating proximal fixation for improved axial stability. The fourth generation of IMF nailing devices are fibular specific and include proximal fixation for improved stability as in the previous generation. They are also differentiated from earlier generations by (1) non-angled syndesmotic slots on the nail/guide to afford syndesmotic realignment along the centroidal axis, and (2) headless interlocking screws to engage the nail itself, rather than cortical bone to mitigate hardware loosening in bone with reduced density.[16] Research over the latest generation of nails is particularly encouraging.[16,17]

Like any new technology and technique, IMF nailing has an initial learning curve and as this method becomes more widely performed, more research and outcome studies will emerge. At this time, IMF nails have been shown to afford equivalent clinical outcomes compared to traditional large incision open reduction internal fixation (ORIF) using plates and screws. Intramedullary fibular nailing also has the benefit for a shorter postoperative convalescence period. Long-term studies that evaluate post-traumatic ankle osteoarthritis after IMF nailing and open plating/screw fixation will be areas for future research. Nonetheless, gaining proficiency with this emerging minimal incision approach to ankle fractures is a necessary skill for the foot and ankle surgeon.

Surgical Technique

The senior authors preferred technique for arthroscopy-assisted ORIF using an IMF nail, with "direct" reduction and syndesmotic realignment along the centroidal axis using a fourth generation IMF nail has been previously published.[16] "Direct" over "Indirect" reduction of the syndesmosis is preferred to avoid the inherent variability associated with tenaculum's/clamps.[18,19] For the operative ankle fracture, the authors advocate preoperative computed tomography to assess any syndesmosis injury, and if a posterior malleolus fracture is present to additionally assess the morphology as well as the presence of any intercalary fragment(s). Ankle arthroscopy is first performed in all cases to lavage the joint of proinflammatory cytokines and fracture hematoma, assess for osteochondral lesions of the talus/tibia, and discern the presence/absence of syndesmotic instability. If non-invasive ankle distraction is utilized, the distractor is released prior to assessment of the syndesmosis to prevent any ligamentous tension distally from causing a false-negative assessment; gravity distraction is preferred.

Following arthroscopy, the sequence for malleolar fracture reduction/fixation is performed in the following order: posterior, medial, and lateral. Intercalary fragments must be excised prior to posterior malleolus fracture fixation. Isolated fractures involving the posterior-lateral tibia plafond are fixated with a single screw placed from posterior to anterior, while those involving the posterior lateral and medial tibial plafond are plated through a posterolateral/posteromedial approach. Medial malleolar fractures involving the anterior colliculus are secured with a single 4.0-mm screw, 45 mm in length, while those involving the entire malleolus are plated.

After fixation of posterior and medial malleolar fractures, the fibula's length, rotation, and angulation are restored using a Hintermann distractor, point-to-point reduction clamp(s), or a combination thereof (**Fig. 1**). When using a distractor, care must be taken to place the K-wires as close as possible on opposing ends of fracture, with placement directed toward either the anterior or posterior half of the fibula. The placement maintains room for the entry wire (diamond or trocar tipped) of the IMF to pass posteriorly or anteriorly, respectively (**Fig. 2**). After initial placement of the IMF, the limb is internally rotated to the "Center-Center" position and the holes are aligned neutrally by rotating the nail (**Fig. 3**). While maintaining the position, the out-rigger guide is then attached; the syndesmosis is manually reduced and held by 2 provisional pins. The pins are placed into the syndesmotic stabilization sots across the fibula and tibia, and maintain the rotation of the IMF, as well as the syndesmosis realignment. Syndesmotic reduction is verified by extending the anterior-lateral portal of the ankle arthroscopy incision 1 to 2 cm proximal, for direct palpation of distal tibiofibular congruence, or through direct visualization of the congruence between the anterolateral tibia and

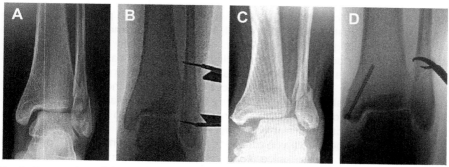

Fig. 1. Restoration of the length, rotation, and angulation of the fibula using a (*A, B*) Hintermann distractor, or (*C, D*) point-to-point reduction clamp.

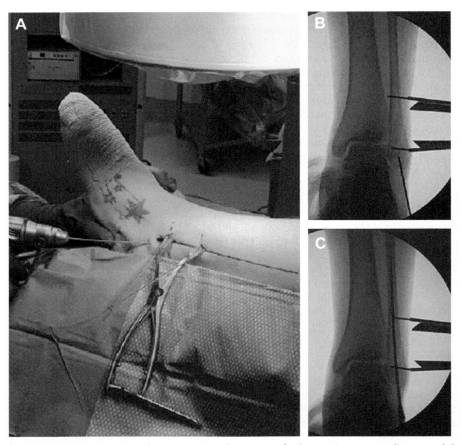

Fig. 2. Intraoperative series demonstrating placement of a large Hintermann distractor (*A*) and introduction of the intramedullary fibular (IMF) nail guidewire (*B, C*). The Hinterman should be placed with closed arms in the anterior or posterior half of the fibula to allow un-obstructed space for the insertion of the IMF nail. For guidewire placement, reaming, and insertion of the Flex-Thread (Coventus Flower Orthopedics, Horsham PA) IMF nail.

anteromedial fibula. Both techniques avoid difficulties with traditional assessment of iatrogenic malreduction using intraoperative fluoroscopy. Two polyaxial screws are then inserted and seated flush with the nail, followed by placement of 2 syndesmotic fixation devices along the centroidal axis. Type of fixation for the syndesmosis is determined at the discretion of the operating surgeon; most cases involve insertion of 2 flexible fixation devices. The most distal fixation was always placed first, followed by fixation proximally. The end result, in most cases, is 4 stab incisions for the lateral malleolus, a single stab incision each for the posterior and medial malleolus, and 2 in-cisions for ankle arthroscopy. This results in a total of 6 to 8 stab incisions, depending on the number of fractures morphology (**Fig. 4**).

Postoperatively, toe-touch weightbearing is permitted immediately, protected weightbearing in a controlled ankle motion boot at 2 weeks, and weightbearing as tolerated in an ankle brace at 6 weeks. Formal physical therapy is commenced at 8 weeks postoperatively.

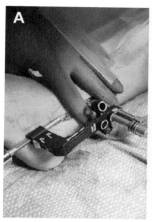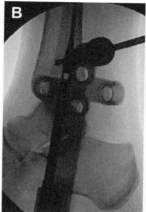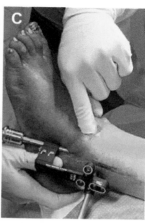

Fig. 3. Intraoperative series demonstrating placement of the IMF nail. The limb is internally rotated (*A*) to achieve "Center-Center" position on intraoperative fluoroscopy (*B*) with the fibula alignment being centrally within the tibia. While holding the limb, the IMF nail itself is then rotated until the syndesmotic holes are perfectly aligned, and the outrigger guide is attached. This position is maintained with 2 provisional K-wire fixation. Syndesmotic realignment (*C*) is then verified by direct palpation of the distal tibiofibular congruence anteriorly. This technique avoids the inherent subjectivity and difficulties associated with intraoperative assessment of syndesmotic alignment.

MINIMALLY INVASIVE PERCUTANEOUS OSTEOSYNTHESIS PLATING

The minimally invasive percutaneous osteosynthesis (MIPO) plating was a method originally described by Brunner and Weber in the 1980s for femoral plating. The MIPO method of plating was later adopted for the tibia (and fibula) and affords buttressing of a fracture through a small soft tissue window, while preserving the native biology with the avoidance of soft tissue striping.[20–22] According to Arbeitsgemeinschaft für Osteosynthesefragen (AO) philosophy, MIPO plating results in reduced surgical trauma, lower infection rates, faster case time, improved recovery time, and preservation of the biology in and around the fracture site. Literature comparing MIPO plating versus ORIF has shown faster healing, with lower infection and reoperation rates in favor of MIPO.

Marazzi and colleagues performed a comparative study between MIPO plating versus ORIF for Wb B and C type fractures, concluding that MIPO was superior in terms of overall complication rates.[23,24] They also noted that MIPO plating resulted in a significant shorter average operative time. Cadaveric study by Kritsaneephaiboon and colleagues evaluating the posterolateral approach for the distal tibial fracture cautions for reduced stability in the sagittal plane, potentially lending the technique prone to procurvatum/recurvatum deformity.[22]

Minimally invasive percutaneous plating for the ankle fracture has the clear benefit of reducing additional soft tissue damage to an already compromised area. The MIPO plating technique is widely accepted, and surgeons should strongly consider this approach. As experience with fracture repair through limited incisions, surgeons will gain more proficiency in treating more complex fractures. Surgeons can additionally gain experience with MIPO by performing it on fifth metatarsal fractures. Nonetheless, each ankle fracture pattern and patient will have its own unique set of indications.

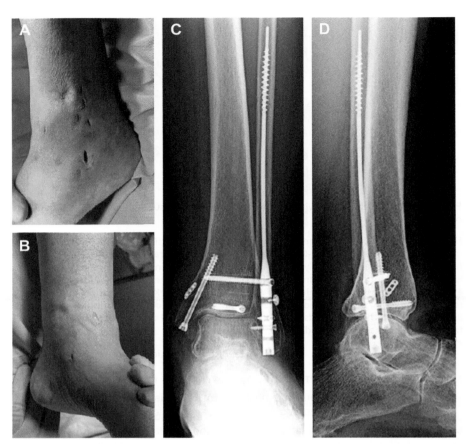

Fig. 4. Trimalleolar ankle fracture repaired with minimally invasive approach with percutaneous screw insertion for the medial malleolus fracture and an IMF nail (Flex-Thread | Coventus Flower Orthopedics, Horsham PA) for the fibular facture. Percutaneous "stab" incisional placement for hardware is demonstrated lateral (*A*) and medially (*B*). Postoperative weight-bearing radiographs (*C, D*) depicting primary healing of a fixated ankle fracture.

Surgical Technique

When considering MIPO plating, preoperative planning is essential as each fracture must be evaluated separately to assess for the ability to buttress the fracture(s). In general, transverse or short oblique fractures in the metaphysis and diaphysis are fixated utilizing the MIPO compression plating technique as those fracture patterns require absolute stability for healing purposes. Bridging comminuted fractures can also be considered. According to a study by Gülabi and colleagues, MIPO plating was best indicated in AO/OTA type A and B fractures.[21]

For tibial fractures, the patient is placed a supine position on the operative table with a bump under the ipsilateral hip to prevent excessive external rotation of the limb. A thigh tourniquet may be applied. Intraoperative fluoroscopy is necessary when utilizing MIPO technique. Some surgeons have recommended tracing the medial malleolus, posterior, and anterior aspects of the tibia at this time with a sterile skin marker since the surgery will be performed with limited incisions.

Reduction of the fracture can be achieved using various methodologies: point-to-point reduction clamp, manual distraction, external fixator/external distractor, and/or push-pull techniques. Once reduction is achieved and confirmed on intra-operative fluoroscopy, a proper plate is selected. According to AO, 3 to 4 screws on either side of the fracture site are suitable for stable MIPO fixation. Anatomically shaped plates versus straight plating should be considered based on the fracture pattern, available real estate, and surgeon's experience. The authors prefer anatomical plates, particularly when considering sliding the plates under the skin. Regarding plate thickness's, 3.5-mm straight (vs 4.5-mm anatomic) is selected when intraoperative contouring is desired. For the tibia, intraoperative contouring should include a 20-degree internal torsion at the distal aspect of the plate to match the anatomy of the tibial bone. Anatomic plates are more often bulky (4.5-mm) as they provide more rigidity; however, they offer little in ways of contouring and can be prominent on the patient's leg and ankle.

After plate selection, the surgeon will make, at minimum, 2 soft tissue windows down to the level of bone. An incision is needed both proximal and distal to the fracture site. The distal incision can be made to the surgeons' preference, but it is generally placed 3 to 4 cm above the level of the ankle joint extending to the medial malleolus, in a curvilinear or straight orientation. The medial anatomic considerations are the saphenous vein and nerve. This soft tissue window will allow the surgeon to have access to the distalmost holes in the plate. At this time, the surgeon can consider using a subcutaneous tunneling device to create a path for the plate to follow on its trek up the tibia. The plate is then inserted into the distal incision and advanced up the tibia; once the plate is in proper position, intra-operative fluoroscopy is used to determine adequate alignment and reduction.

The proximal incision may be created either before the insertion of the compression plate or afterward. This incision is placed on the medial proximal portion of the tibial diaphysis. The incision should allow the surgeon to visualize the plate's proximal screw holes. Once reduction and plate placement are confirmed, an antiglide screw is placed bicortically in the distal aspect of the plate to prevent vertical shear, depending on the fracture pattern. This initial screw must be placed bicortically, and a longer-than-necessary screw can be deployed that will be exchanged later in the procedure. Following this primary screw placement, if the fracture pattern permits, a screw can be placed through the site of the fracture. A stab incision or minimal incision can be made overlying the area of the plate that is adjacent to the fracture where the intra-fracture screw can be placed. For added compression, an eccentrically drilled screw can be inserted proximal to the fracture site.

Surgeons have described a lag screw through the plate, across the fracture site. However, it should be noted that depending on the fracture pattern, a lag screw may not be permissible through the plate. In some cases, an additional stab incision must be made to insert an interfrag screw as perpendicularly as possible through the fracture site off of the plate. Finally, the surgeon can complete fixation by inserting an adequate number of screws (3–4 distal and proximal). Fewer screws are required through the diaphyseal portion of the bone for adequate fixation. The aforementioned description is of MIPO plating the medial aspect of the tibia which is preferable. However, lateral tibial plating can be necessary when medial soft tissue is damaged or the fracture pattern requires it.

The lateral incisions are made distally in the interval between the deep peroneal nerve and superficial peroneal nerve, care must be taken to avoid anterior neurovascular bundle in this area. Deep dissection will allow identification of the anterior tibial tendon which should be retracted laterally along with the deep peroneal nerve and anterior tibial vessels. The proximal incision is made distal from the tibial tubercle and 1.5 to 2 cm lateral to the tibial crest, this incision can be extended distally up to 5 cm. In this window, the anterior tibial muscle can be identified and this will be retracted laterally.

For fibular MIPO plating, 2 soft tissue windows are created, and possibly an additional stab incision to place a lag screw perpendicular through the fracture site. If placing a lag screw through a percutaneous stab incision, do so initially after achieving adequate reduction. Following this, the minimally invasive plate will be applied. A 2 cm long incision is made distally overlying the fibula. This incision should incorporate the distal-most end of the fibula. A fibular plate will be selected and inserted in this distal soft tissue window. A locking tower can be placed on the distal end of the plate to have leverage when retrograding the plate. Once reduction and position of the plate is confirmed through intra-operative fluoroscopy, an additional 2 to 3 cm incision can be made overlying the proximal portion of the plate. A locking tower can be placed on the proximal most end of the plate, utilizing this and the distal locking tower, the plate can be moved easier through the frontal plane for adequate placement. Once the plate is in the most desirable position, the plate holes are filled with locking screws proximal and distal to the fracture site.

TRANSPORTAL RETROGRADE TIBIOTALOCALCANEAL ARTHRODESIS

The role of TibioTaloCalcaneal (TTC) nailing plays an important role in the realm of foot and ankle surgery, particularly for combined hindfoot and ankle arthrosis. Moreso, the TTC nail is often performed with Charcot arthropathy reconstruction for the ability to provide a rigid limb for the patient to ambulate on.[25–28] In trauma involving the geriatric and/or severely comminuted injuries, fusion of the anke and subtalar joint is often a viable option. Neuropathic ankle fractures have significant postoperative sequela with traditional open approaches and percutaneous TTC nailing is an ideal solution in some patients (**Fig. 5**).

Complications of TTC nailing include hardware failure, nonunion, and infections. In order to mitigate possible complications, transportal/arthroscopic joint preparation of the ankle and subtalar joints has been described.[29] Performing arthroscopic joint preparation during TTC cases allows minimal soft tissue exposure, affords the same level of joint preparation, and in the hands of a well-versed physician can also decrease total operative time, which is directly correlated to postoperative infection.[30–32]

Baumbach and colleagues demonstrated in their study that arthroscopic joint preparation, as opposed to open, drastically reduced surgical site infections.[25] Similarly, Younger and colleagues compared open versus arthroscopic TTC as well. Their study showed that arthroscopic TTC arthrodesis had lower non-union rates and lower infections rates, along with no reoperation rates as opposed to the open TTC fusion group.[32]

Of course, as with any approach, careful consideration must be taken by the surgeon when employing arthroscopic joint preparation for TTC nailing. One of the most important considerations would be level of deformity in the rearfoot. Though arthroscopic debridement of the cartilage allows adequate joint preparation, often indications for a TTC involve complex planal deformities in the rearfoot. Arthroscopic joint preparation will provide the surgeon minimum in terms of complex deformity correction.

Pushing the envelope further in terms of TTC nailing will require the ability to correct deformities through percutaneous approaches. Granted, for complex rigid

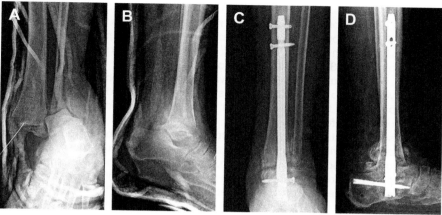

Fig. 5. Open dislocated trimalleolar ankle fracture (*A, B*) in an uncontrolled diabetic patient with peripheral neuropathy treated with primary arthrodesis with transportal retrograde tibiotalocalcaneal arthrodesis (*C, D*). A stable pseudoarthrosis at 12-months postoperatively with well aligned limb.

deformities, open correction will likely remain the gold standard. For now, there seems to be consensus in literature that arthroscopic joint preparation provides benefits in terms of limiting post operative complications, improving time to heal/union, and decreasing operating time. There is still a paucity of literature on this topic and an area for future research studies to emerge.

Surgical Technique

The basic principles of TTC arthrodesis with a nail involve adequate joint preparation of the ankle and subtalar joint, correction of deformity if one presents, and application of the nail with the foot externally rotated 5 to 10° and in either neutral or up to 5° of valgus. There are a myriad of hardware companies that have different techniques of nail preparation, but the insertion of the TTC nail follows the same algorithm: stab incision to the plantar aspect of the heel, guide wire insertion through the calcaneus, talus, and into the tibial canal, drilling over the guide wire, reaming, and lastly nail insertion.

Care must be taken when inserting the hindfoot nail as damage to the lateral plantar artery, nerve, and Baxter's nerve can occur. Belcyzk and colleagues in 2008 did describe a method to best avoid the neurovascular bundle and also provided a guide for adequate placement of the rearfoot nail.[26] For this method, the practitioner will utilize intra-operative fluoroscopy. The guide wire is placed laterally on the patient's leg, and under radiography, the wire is approximated to the central tibial canal. Once this position is found, a line is drawn on the patient's leg. The guide wire should be bisecting the lateral talar process. This line is traced down to the foot and continued on the plantar aspect. Next, a calcaneal axial is taken with a Schanz pin, or equally robust pin, bisecting the calcaneus. Once this position is found, a vertical line is drawn and this line should be perpendicular to the first line. The intersection of these lines is the ideal position for the nail insertion. Note, that the surgeon must medialize the talus and calcaneus on the tibia in order to align the rearfoot in the best position.

Prior to the advent of arthroscopic debridement of cartilage, resection of the subtalar and ankle joints was performed with large incisions to access both joints. In some cases, the fibula is osteotomized and/or removed entirely. There are variations in the literature as to what should be done with fibula during this procedure. Wu and colleagues in 2020 performed TTC in 155 ankles, with 94 ankles in the fibula-spared group and 61 in the fibular resection group. The results showed no difference in healing time and time to union for either group.[31] However, in 2023, a study by He and colleagues comparing 3 different groups of TTC with fibular procedures: fibular osteotomy, fibular strut, and fibular preservation revealed that the fibular strut group had improved time to union. The fibular strut group consisted of the fibula being resected; one-half of the fibula was used as an autograft, and the other half was used as an on lay graft.[28]

Though some literature exists, there is still debate as to the best procedure to be done to the fibula during TTC nailing. Once arthroscopy was introduced, there presented a novel method of joint preparation. With this method, however, the fibula is generally spared to allow minimally invasive nail application. Anteromedial and anterolateral ankle portals are most often employed via stab incisions. The anteromedial incision is placed medial to the tibialis anterior tendon and lateral to medial malleolus with care to avoid the saphenous nerve in this area. The anterolateral incision is made medial to the lateral malleolus and lateral to the peroneus tertius, this is where the superficial peroneal nerve can be found. The posterior ankle portals can also be used if the patient must be placed in a prone position. With respect to the subtalar joint, the 2 portals most often employed are the dorsolateral portal and the posterolateral portal. The dorsolateral portal is located at the junction between the talonavicular and calcaneocuboid joints and the posterolateral portal is located at the lateral side of the Achilles tendon (about 2 cm posterior and 1 cm proximal to the fibular tip).

Once access is gained to the ankle and subtalar joints, the cartilage is debrided, the foot is positioned adequately, and then the nail is implanted. The purpose of arthroscopic joint preparation is to pay as much respect possible to the soft tissue and in turn attempting to increase healing/union time. A systematic review by Lameire and colleagues in 2023 reviewed 5 articles, 4 of which arthroscopic debridement was performed for TTC nailing. The results proved favorable in terms of healing/union time and low complication rates. For now, the arthroscopic approach to joint preparation during TTC nailing remains a viable option.[29]

CALCANEAL FRACTURE

Calcaneal fractures represent 2% of foot and ankle trauma. These fractures typically occur due to an axial load from falling from a height or high-energy trauma. Approximately 60% to 75% of calcaneal fractures are displaced intra-articular fractures.[33,34] Studies have shown that surgical treatment of intra-articular calcaneal fractures improves functional outcomes and patient satisfaction when compared to conservative treatment. However, the fixation and surgical approach of intra-articular calcaneal fractures remains a topic of current debate.

Open extensile approaches of the calcaneal fracture have been mainstream due to the exceptional visualization, ability to visually anatomically reduce the fracture(s) with buttress plating. However, this widely open approach is risky for would dehiscence and subsequent osteomyelitis. With the rise of minimally invasive surgery, the treatment of the calcaneal fracture has become a viable approach that offers the potential for reduced soft tissue trauma, adequate visualization, and expedited recovery (**Fig. 6**).

Current literature presents similar results when minimally invasive techniques are used for the treatment of calcaneal fractures, with low incidence of soft tissue complications, good functional outcomes, less trauma, and reduced blood loss, when

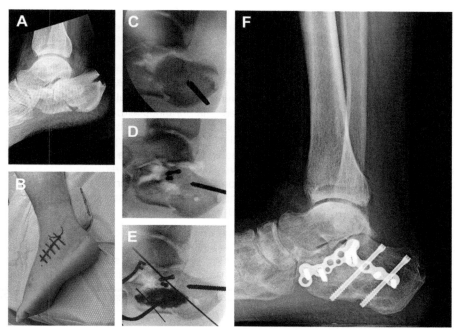

Fig. 6. Minimal incision repair of displaced tongue type calcaneal fracture. Preoperative radiograph (*A*). Intraoperative image illustrating incision placement (*B*). Intraoperative fluoroscopic series illustrating reduction (*C*), posterior facet fixation, (*D*) and allograft placement (*E*). Final healed radiographs at 12-weeks (*F*).

compared to extensive open reduction. A retrospective study by DeWall and colleagues demonstrated no significant differences in the Böhler angle values between the minimally invasive and open reduction techniques for displaced intra-articular calcaneal fractures.[35] Additionally, the infection rates were lower in patients who were treated using the minimally invasive technique, suggesting that this technique was superior with respect to lower complication rates and improved functional result. Kline and colleagues (2013) compared the extensile lateral approach to a minimally invasive approach in 125 intra-articular calcaneal fractures and found that the minimally invasive approach minimized complications, achieved and maintained extra-articular reductions as well as the standard extensile open approach.[36]

The minimal incision approach for calcaneal fracture fixation offers another tool for the foot and ankle surgeon. The fracture pattern must be taken into careful consideration when considering this approach. If employed, however, positive results have been seen and lower postoperative complication rates are reported.

Surgical Technique

The patient is positioned on their side in lateral decubitus with the knee flexed at 90° for the minimally invasive treatment of intra-articular calcaneal fractures. A 5-cm skin incision is started just below the tip of the lateral malleolus in line with the posterior malleolar cortex toward the base of the fourth metatarsal. Subperiosteal blunt dissection of the lateral wall is performed using a large cobb. Care should be taken to dissect the peroneal tendons and keep the peroneal sheath intact. Care should also be taken to avoid injury to either the superficial peroneal or sural nerves. The sinus tarsi fat pad is excised. The collapsed posterior facet of the calcaneus is elevated to obtain anatomic subtalar joint reduction and percutaneously fixated using K-wires. A trans calcaneal shanz pin is used to correct for varus and valgus of the calcaneal tuberosity. Stabilization of the reduction is temporarily fixated with percutaneous screws, K-wires, Steinman pins, or a combination therein. Large defects after reduction are filled with autograft/allograft and then fixated with an appropriate size anatomic plate. The plate is inserted into the interval between the peroneus tendon and lateral wall of the calcaneus. Supplementary screws may be placed for ancillary tongue type fracture patterns, or additional stability.[35–37]

Final position is confirmed on fluoroscopy and a drainage tube is placed in situ. The sutures are removed 2 weeks post operatively and the patient is remained non-weight bearing until radiographic signs of bony consolidation are observed.

SUMMARY

Minimally invasive surgery, particularly in the trauma setting, reduces the risk of soft tissue complications and SSI. Although the learning curve is steep and the initial cost of implants may be higher compared to traditional open surgery, the reduced complication rates result in better quality of care, and an overall lower cost of health care delivery. In the current era of increasing cost containment and reimbursements tied to "outcome," the authorsIMF feel it is salient all podiatric surgeons become well versed in the technique(s).

CLINICS CARE POINTS

- Arthroscopy-assisted minimally invasive ankle fracture repair acts as a lavage, eliminating the pro-inflammatory milieu inside the ankle following trauma.
- When performing intramedullary fibular nailing, pin distractors should be positioned in the anterior or posterior half of the fibula, leaving room for insertion of a fibular nail.
- For MIPO plating, the orthopedic hardware selection can be straight plates that are contoured intraoperatively or anatomically shaped plates.
- Neuropathic ankle fractures that are treated with transportal TTC nailing should be manually compressed prior to nail insertion.
- Use of a pin-distractor, clamp, or combination thereof allows for in-direct fracture reduction without traditional incisional exposure(s).

DISCLOSURE

The authors have nothing to disclose.

REFERENCES

1. Belatti DA, Phisitkul P. Economic burden of foot and ankle surgery in the US medicare population. Foot Ankle Int 2014;35(4):334–40.
2. Roukis TS. Bacterial skin contamination before and after surgical preparation of the foot, ankle, and lower leg in patients with diabetes and intact skin versus patients with diabetes and ulceration: a prospective controlled therapeutic study. J Foot Ankle Surg 2010;49(4):348–56.

3. Rushing CJ. Retrospective analysis of operating room irrigation using a low concentration chlorhexidine gluconate (CHG) 0.05% in sterile water for infection prevention after foot & ankle surgery. Foot Ankle Surg: Techniques, Reports Cases 2023;3(1):100264–10266.
4. Hunter JG, Dawson LK, Soin SP, et al. Randomized, prospective study of the order of preoperative preparation solutions for patients undergoing foot and ankle orthopedic surgery. Foot Ankle Int 2016;37(5):478–82.
5. Kleinert JM, Hoffmann J, Miller Crain G, et al. Postoperative infection in a double-occupancy operating room. A prospective study of two thousand four hundred and fifty-eight procedures on the extremities. J Bone Joint Surg Am 1997;79(4):503–13.
6. Contreras ES, Frantz TL, Bishop JY, et al. Periprosthetic infection after reverse shoulder arthroplasty: a review. Curr Rev Musculoskelet Med 2020;6:757–68.
7. Gold PA, Garbarino LJ, Sodhi N, et al. A 6-year trends analysis of infections after revision total hip arthroplasty. Ann Transl Med 2019;7(4):76.
8. Thompson O, W-Dahl A, Lindgren V, et al. Similar periprosthetic joint infection rates after and before a national infection control program: a study of 45,438 primary total knee arthroplasties. Acta Orthop 2021;17:1–7.
9. Carl J, Shelton TJ, Nguyen K, et al. Effect of postoperative oral antibiotics on infections and wound healing following foot and ankle surgery. Foot Ankle Int 2020;41(12):1466–73.
10. Williamson DA, Carter GP, Howden BP. Current and emerging topical antibacterials and antiseptics: agents, action, and resistance patterns. Clin Microbiol Rev 2017;30(3):827–60.
11. Lynde MJ, Sautter T, Hamilton GA, et al. Complications after open reduction and internal fixation of ankle fractures in the elderly. Foot Ankle Surg 2012;18(2):103–7.
12. Jain S, Haughton BA, Brew C. Intramedullary fixation of distal fibular fractures: a systematic review of clinical and functional outcomes. J Orthop Traumatol 2014;15(4):245–54.
13. Jordan RW, Chapman AWP, Buchanan D, et al. The role of intramedullary fixation in ankle fractures - a systematic review. Foot Ankle Surg 2018;24(1):1–10.
14. Tas DB, Smeeing DPJ, Emmink BL, et al. Intramedullary fixation versus plate fixation of distal fibular fractures: a systematic review and meta-analysis of randomized controlled trials and observational studies. J Foot Ankle Surg 2019;58(1):119–26.
15. Raj V, Barik S, Richa. Distal fibula fractures-intramedullary fixation versus plating: a systematic review and meta-analysis of randomized control trials. Foot Ankle Spec 2022. https://doi.org/10.1177/19386400221118470.
16. Rushing CJ. Comparison of ankle fracture fixation using an intramedullary fibular nail versus plate fixation. J Foot Ankle Surg 2024;63(5):546–56.
17. Rushing CJ. Ankle fracture reduction using A novel, flexible intramedullary fibular nail and alignment guide affording syndesmotic Re-alignment along the centroidal Axis. Foot Ankle Surg, Techniques, Reports Cases 2023;3(4). https://doi.org/10.1016/j.fastrc.2023.100271.
18. Rushing CJ, Spinner SM, Armstrong AV, et al. Comparison of different magnitudes of applied syndesmotic clamp force: a cadaveric study. J Foot Ankle Surg 2020;59(3):452–6.
19. Rushing CJ, Spinner SM, Armstrong AV, et al. Proximal placement of the syndesmotic reduction clamp and the optimal position for the medial tine. A cadaveric pilot study. J Foot Ankle Surg 2022;61(1):3–6.

20. Barış A, Çirci E, Demirci Z, et al. Minimally invasive medial plate osteosynthesis in tibial pilon fractures: longterm functional and radiological outcomes. Acta Orthop Traumatol Turc 2020;54(1):20–6.
21. Gülabi D, Bekler Hİ, Sağlam F, et al. Surgical treatment of distal tibia fractures: open versus MIPO. Ulus Travma Acil Cerrahi Derg 2016;22(1):52–7.
22. Kritsaneephaiboon A, Vaseenon T, Tangtrakulwanich B. Minimally invasive plate osteosynthesis of distal tibial fracture using a posterolateral approach: a cadaveric study and preliminary report. Int Orthop 2013;37(1):105–11.
23. Marazzi C, Wittauer M, Hirschmann MT, et al. Minimally invasive plate osteosynthesis (MIPO) versus open reduction and internal fixation (ORIF) in the treatment of distal fibula Danis-Weber types B and C fractures. J Orthop Surg Res 2020; 15(1):49.
24. Park YJ, Hwang Y, Shim D-W, et al. Treatment of 5th metatarsal shaft fracture using MIPO (minimally invasive plate osteosynthesis) technique. Foot Ankle Orthopaedics 2017;2(3). https://doi.org/10.1177/2473011417S000318.
25. Baumbach SF, Massen FK, Hörterer S, et al. Comparison of arthroscopic to open tibiotalocalcaneal arthrodesis in high-risk patients. Foot Ankle Surg 2019;25(6): 804–11.
26. Belczyk RJ, Sung W, Wukich DK. Technical tip: a simple method for proper placement of an intramedullary nail entry point for tibiotalocalcaneal or tibiocalcaneal arthrodesis. Foot Ankle J 2008. https://doi.org/10.3827/faoj.2008.0109.0004.
27. de Cesar Netto C, Johannesmeyer D, Cone B, et al. Neurovascular structures at risk with curved retrograde TTC fusion nails. Foot Ankle Int 2017;38(10):1139–45.
28. He W, Zhou H, Li Z, et al. Comparison of different fibula procedures in tibiotalocalcaneal arthrodesis with a retrograde intramedullary nail: a mid-term retrospective study. BMC Muscoskel Disord 2023;24(1):882.
29. Lameire DL, Abdel Khalik H, Del Balso C, et al. Transportal tibiotalocalcaneal nail ankle arthrodesis: a systematic review of initial series. Foot Ankle Orthop 2023; 8(1). 24730114231156422.
30. Scigliano NM, Carender CN, Glass NA, et al. Operative time and risk of surgical site infection and periprosthetic joint infection: a systematic review and meta-analysis. Iowa Orthop J 2022;42(1):155–61.
31. Wu M, Scott DJ, Schiff AP, et al. Does a fibula-sparing approach improve outcomes in tibiotalocalcaneal arthrodesis? Foot Ankle Orthop 2020;29(1):90–6.
32. Younger AS, Leucht A, Wing K, et al. Podium presentation title: arthroscopic vs. Open combined ankle and subtalar fusion using a retrograde tibial nail. Arthroscopy 2023;39(6):1 e14–e15.
33. Bajammal S, Tornetta PR, Sanders D, et al. Displaced intra-articular calcaneal fractures. J Orthop Trauma 2005;19:360–4.
34. Cursaru A, Crețu B, Șerban B, et al. Minimally invasive treatment and internal fixation vs. extended lateral approach in calcaneus fractures of thalamic interest. Exp Ther Med 2022;23(3):196.
35. DeWall M, Henderson CE, McKinley TO, et al. Percutaneous reduction and fixation of displaced intra-articular calcaneus fractures. J Orthop Trauma 2010;24: 466–72.
36. Kline AJ, Anderson RB, Davis WH, et al. Minimally invasive technique versus an extensile lateral approach for intra-articular calcaneal fractures. Foot Ankle Int 2013;34:773–80.
37. Potter MQ, Nunley JA. Long-term functional outcomes after operative treatment for intra-articular fractures of the calcaneus. J Bone Joint Surg Am 2009;91: 1854–60.

Controversial Matters of Minimally Invasive Bunion Repair

Gustavo Araujo Nunes, MD, PhD(c)[a],*,
Francisco Sánchez Villanueva, MD[b],
Felipe Chaparro Ravazzano, MD[c], Tiago Baumfeld, MD, PhD[d]

KEYWORDS

- Minimally invasive bunion surgery • Percutaneous surgery • Hallux valgus • Bunion

KEY POINTS

- Despite recent advances in minimally invasive bunion surgery (MIBS) for treating hallux valgus (HV), there are controversial matters that should be discussed and studied.
- First-ray hypermobility and rotational correction of HV are controversial issues in MIBS, similar to those in open surgery.
- The controversies linked to the MIS technique are related to the shape of the osteotomy and the use, configuration, and quantity of screws used to stabilize the osteotomies.

INTRODUCTION

In the last decade there has been a significant push for biomechanical studies and refinement of surgical techniques related to new minimally invasive bunion surgery (MIBS). The adoption of minimally invasive (MI) techniques as a mainstay treatment in hallux valgus (HV) surgery is supported by growing and robust literature.[1,2] MIBS has evolved through a better understanding of the anatomy, improvements in MI instruments, implant (MI screw) advancements and the technique refinements. The development of the MI screw fixated osteotomies has made this approach more reproducible and predictable.[3,4]

The first version (or generation) of MIBS was the unfixated Reverdin-Isham osteotomy. The second-generation MIBS involved the percutaneous K-wire fixation of a subcapital osteotomy. The next MIBS generation involves two percutaneous MI screw

[a] Foot and Ankle Unit, COTE Brasília Clinic, Federal District, Brazil; [b] Department of Orthopedic Surgery, Foot and Ankle Center, Clínica Puerto Varas y Puerto Montt, Chile; [c] Department of Orthopedic Surgery, Foot and Ankle Center, Clínica Universidad de los Andes, Chile; [d] Foot and Ankle Unit, Hospital Felício Rocho, Belo Horizonte, Minas Gerais, Brazil
* Corresponding author. SGAS 915 Lote 68a Salas 16/17 Centro Clínico Advance 2 - Asa Sul, Brasília - DF 70390-150, Brazil.
E-mail address: gustavoanunes@hotmail.com

fixation with a chevron ostetomy developed by Redfern and Vernois. A slight variation in the osteotomy configuration to a transverse osteotomy has led some to call this a fourth generation MIBS.[5,6] Recently introduced (Blitz 2023) is fifth and sixth generation MIBS that involve a single metatarsal screw construct paired with a stabilizing osteotomy, and is discussed later in the chapter. Practically speaking, "new" MIBS refers to a percutaneous subcapital osteotomy fixated with MI screw(s). The most studied version of MIBS is the chevron osteotomy and two metatarsal screw construct involving a wide variety of bunion severities has made this the most currently accepted method/construct.[1,4,5]

HV is a complex deformity with over a hundred different surgical operations described. With new MIBS emerging as the dominant surgical treatment for bunions, there are many controversial aspects that have emerged as topic of worldwide debate.[7,8] Newer publications are aimed at dispelling myths or providing supportive evidence that further positions MIBS as the gold standard for bunion surgery.[6,9–13] Traditionalists remain vocal that MI may not be better than open surgery as it relates to long-term results.[1,14]

Some of the pivotal controversial matters of MIBS are similar to those of open bunion surgery. The most polemic ones are how to address first-ray hypermobility and protonation.[7,9,10] Both subjects demand further assessment, preoperative planning, and intraoperative control to better correct the deformity. Another important controversy surrounds the technical aspect of the osteotomy configuration and what is the optimal fixation construct/type.[3,15,16] While the chevron subcapital osteotomy was the first described, it has some rotational constraints questioning its "superiority."[6,9] And, despite MI bunion surgery classically being performed worldwide sans fixation, controversy and disagreement exists surrounding the optimal MI screw fixation quantity, type and/or construct.[17,18]

CONTROVERSY 1: IS OPEN SURGERY SUPERIOR TO MINIMALLY INVASIVE BUNION SURGERY?

The traditional approach to HV correction involves medium-to-large incisions on the dorsum or side of the bunion and/or the entire first ray. Open surgery has the obvious benefit of direct visualization of the osseous anatomy for the reduction of deformity and the delivery of surgical hardware/implants. Traditional chevron osteotomies were performed open and located within the metaphyseal section of the metatarsal head. The popular scarf osteotomy was also performed via a direct visualization approach through expansile linear incisions. Numerous studies have reported satisfactory outcomes with open surgery, demonstrating significant improvements in pain, function, and alignment. One particular study by Molloy and Widnall[19] showed a mean American Orthopaedic Foot & Ankle Society hallux metatarsophalangeal–interphalangeal scale score improvement from 53.5 to 91.1 following open correction procedures. Open surgery is associated with several drawbacks that include wound complications (due to the larger incisions and soft tissue trauma) and delayed healing. Extensive dissection may lead to postoperative scar development, stiffness, and prolonged recovery times.[20]

MIBS aims to achieve correction through small incisions using specialized instrumentation and implants (MI screws) with precise fluoroscopic guidance. Several studies have demonstrated favorable outcomes with MI techniques, highlighting reduced postoperative pain, quicker recovery, and improved cosmesis compared to open surgery. A meta analysis by Song and colleagues[21] reported significantly lower visual analog scale pain scores and shorter time to return to regular shoes in patients undergoing MI surgery compared to open surgery. A more recent meta-analyses made by Ji and colleagues[1] involved 22 MI surgery clinical and radiographic studies with over 1500 feet, concluded that MI procedures were more effective (better outcomes) than open surgeries in treating HV. A MIBS become more widely adopted additional studies that will add to the body of evidence on the efficacy of MIBS, and likely the new gold standard for bunion surgery.

CONTROVERSY 2: CAN MINIMALLY INVASIVE BUNION SURGERY CORRECT FRONTAL PLANE ROTATION?

HV is a multi-planar deformity and therefore the pronation (frontal plane) must be considered when correcting the deformity. Many authors opine that frontal plane deformity must be specifically corrected otherwise postoperative bunion recurrence may ensue.[22–24] Frontal plane rotation has been specifically targeted with various open surgery techniques that include the proximal oblique sliding closing wedge osteotomy, proximal metatarsal dome osteotomy, Lapidus arthrodesis, and proximal rotational metatarsal osteotomy.[25–27]

New MIBS can also adequately address frontal plane rotation. While the chevron-subcapital osteotomy frontal plane correction is locked into the osteotomy configuration, the transverse-subcapital osteotomy allows for full rotatory adjustments of the capital fragment, allowing surgeons to subjectively dial in the final frontal plane position. The exact amount of frontal plane correction is determined by the surgeons and studies are lacking as to whether frontal plane correction is associated with improved MIBS results.[6,10]

In attempt to reproducibly "dial in or control" frontal plane rotational correction, the authors (G.N. and T.G.) developed an external fixation device to assist in the correction[9] (**Fig. 1**). The first modification of MIBS to directly address pronation was published by Nunes and Baumfeld.[9] Assesing the preoperative pronation/frontal plane to be corrected may be performed through weightbearing computed tomography or with a weightbearing sesamoidal axial radiopgraph view. The goal is to know the pronation to be corrected preoperativelly and to have a quantitative control intraoperativelly (**Fig. 2**).[28,29]

CONTROVERSY 3: IS FIXATION NECESSARY FOR MINIMALLY INVASIVE BUNION SURGERY?

MI has revolutionized the surgical management of HV, offering reduced soft tissue trauma, faster recovery, and improved cosmetic outcomes compared to traditional

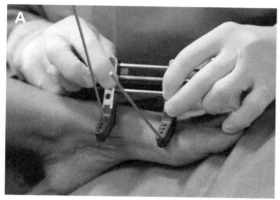
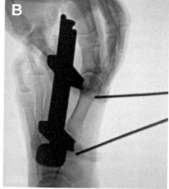

Fig. 1. (*A*) Clinical and (*B*) fluoroscopic image of the rotational correction guide.

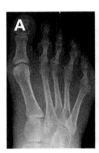 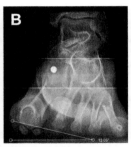 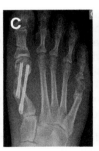 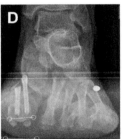

Fig. 2. Radiographic series of a 34 years old female who inderwent a transverse MIBS with rotational correction. Preoperative anteroposterior (A) and weightbearing sesamoid axial view (B) showing a moderate hallux valgus with 13 degrees of metatarsal pronation angle. 06 weeks postoperative anteroposterior (A) and weightbearing sesamoid axial view (B) showing a tridimensional deformity correction.

open techniques.[1] However, MIBS can be performed with or without fixation (hardware). The unfixated version of MIBS (first generation-type) involves the Reverdin-Isham that gains its stability from soft tissue tension, osteotomy configuration and extrinsic bandaging.[17] As for fixated MIBS, the current "most popular" version involves the use implanted screw(s) that are designed specifically for this type of bunion correction, where long scaffolding screws hold together bones that are in near discontinuity.[30] Although fixation may favor osteotomy consolidation, some surgeons opt for unfixed percutaneous osteotomy bunion corrections, prompting questions about the necessity of screw fixation in osteotomy healing. Although fixation may favor osteotomy consolidation, some surgeons opt for unfixed percutaneous osteotomy bunion corrections, prompting questions about the necessity of screw fixation in osteotomy healing. The main reason for internal fixation is to stabilize (or maintain correction/position) the bones for bone healing (first metatarsal regeneration, FMR) during the postoperative period.[12]

Fixation with Minimally Invasive Bunion Surgery: Advantages and Disadvantages

Advantages

1. Enhanced stability: Fixation devices provide immediate stability, reducing the risk of postoperative displacement or loss of correction.
2. Improved precision: Fixation facilitates precise control over the correction achieved during surgery.
3. Early mobilization: With stable fixation, patients may be allowed to bear weight earlier, potentially accelerating rehabilitation.
4. Reduced risk of recurrence: Secure fixation reduces the likelihood of deformity recurrence by maintaining proper alignment during healing.

Disadvantages

1. Soft tissue irritation: Fixation devices may cause soft tissue irritation, leading to discomfort or the need for hardware removal in some cases.
2. Risk of hardware complications: There is a potential risk of hardware-related complications such as loosening, migration, or breakage.
3. Additional surgical steps: The placement of fixation devices adds complexity to the surgical procedure and may prolong operative time.
4. Cost: The use of fixation devices may increase the overall cost of surgery.

Unfixated Minimally Invasive Bunion Surgery: Advantages and Disadvantages

Advantages

1. Minimized soft tissue trauma: Avoidance of fixation reduces the risk of soft tissue irritation and the potential need for hardware removal.
2. Simplified procedure: Elimination of fixation devices streamlines the surgical technique, potentially reducing operative time.
3. Lower risk of hardware complications: Without fixation, hardware-related complications such as loosening or breakage is not risky.
4. Potentially lower cost: The absence of fixation devices may result in lower overall surgical costs.

Disadvantages

1. Less immediate stability: Without fixation, there may be less immediate stability, increasing the risk of displacement or loss of correction.
2. Limited correction: Complex deformities or significant instability may be challenging to correct adequately without fixation.
3. Delayed recovery: patients usually start mobilizing the hallux later since osteotomies must be stabilized by dressings. This can affect mainly younger patients who need to return to sports earlier.
4. Higher risk of recurrence: The absence of fixation may increase the risk of deformity recurrence during the healing process.

Both MI approaches with and without fixation offer unique advantages and limitations in the surgical management of HV. Fixation provides immediate stability and precise control over correction but entails risks such as hardware complications (ie, failure, infected hardware). On the other hand, approaches without fixation minimize soft tissue trauma and simplify the procedure but may have limitations in achieving and maintaining adequate stability. The choice between these approaches should be individualized based on the patient's specific deformity, surgeon expertise, and preferences, aiming to optimize outcomes while minimizing potential risks.[31] The authors prefer fixated MIBS techniques to achieve an intraoperative corrective osseous position and stability allowing for quick/early mobilization for potentially improved functional result. The literature, however, still lacks direct comparative studies and it is not currently possible to affirm the superiority of fixated MIBS versus unfixated MIBS.

CONTROVERSY 4: DOES MINIMALLY INVASIVE BUNION SURGERY TREAT FIRST-RAY HYPERMOBILITY?

First-ray hypermobility was described as a pathologic increased first-ray mobility that occurs as a consequence of midfoot joint instability, mainly the first tarsometatarsal joint and intercuneiform joints.[32] Controversy surrounds first-ray hypermobility from its mere presence, to how it relates to HV formation and recurrence after bunionectomy. Pathologic first ray hypermobility is subjective, difficult to evaluate, measure, and even quantify.[33] Radiographically first-ray hypermobility is suggested with increased intermetatarsal angle. For the past decade or so, arthrodesis of the first tarsometatarsal joint has been considered the "best" approach to eliminate bunion-related hypermobility. However, non-fusion-based hypermobility treatment exists, and has been an area for investigation. Rush and colleagues[34] in a cadaveric study suggested that hypermobility is quelled through a traditional distal metaphyseal chevron osteotomy by reengaging the windlass mechanism. In contrast, other authors believe that stabilizing first tarsometatarsal joint can be accomplished by realigning distal soft tissues through distal osteotomies.[7,33]

MIBS can also treat hypermobility. The mechanism of first-ray stabilization (aka locking of the first ray) with MIBS was proposed by the senior author (G.N.).[7] In this landmark MIBS study using a subcapital chevron osteotomy, the authors proposed that the increased varus displacement of the proximal fragment (metatarsal) in maximum medial position stabilized the transverse plane and reducing the rate of recurrence[7] (Fig. 3). With severe cases, recurrence rates between MIBS and open midfoot fusion surgery (Lapidus-type bunionectomy). On the other hand, Cody and colleagues[35] showed a comparative study between chevron-osteotomy MIBS and Lapidus. They observed some cases with a progressive medialization of the proximal fragment of the osteotomy with a recurrence of the deformity in the MIBS group.[34]

The authors believe that MIBS can stabilize the first ray and address the majority of the cases of HV with hypermobility. We believe that there is a need for a series of cases with long-term follow-up to analyze the behavior of first tarsometatarsal joint and inter-cuneiform joint after MIBS. The authors currently advocate Lapidus-type fusion (over MIBS) first tarsometatarsal joint arthrosis and/or "severe hypermobility." However, defining severe hypermobility is challenging and it is very possible that MIBS would be suitable for these cases.

In an attempt to make an anecdotally objective decision on whether to fuse, the authors perform a preoperative radiographic squeeze test by manually splaying the first and second metatarsals on a non-weightbearing anteroposterior radiograph (Fig. 4). The surgeon assesses whether 100% of head lateralization with MIBS can cover the first metatarsal space. There are 3 scenarios: (1) metatarsal head > intermetatarsal space; (2) metatarsal head = intermetatarsal space; and (3) metatarsal head < intermetatarsal space. In the first scenario, when the metatarsal head is bigger/wider than the intermetatarsal space then MIBS would be effective as there should adequate bone-to-bone contact. In the second scenario, when the metatarsal head the same size/width as the intermetatarsal space, then there would likely be 100% lateral displacement of the capital fragment to correct the deformity with MIBS. In the third scenario, when the metatarsal head is smaller/narrower than the intermetatarsal space, then there could be over 100% lateral displacement of the capital fragment with MIBS, suggesting a proximal osteotomy or Lapidus-type fusion may be more appropriate (depending on the surgeon's MIBS experience).

CONTROVERSY 5: OSTEOTOMY CONFIGURATION: TRANSVERSE VERSUS CHEVRON

Much of the current literature is based on chevron osteotomy MIBS, which has been well established as the predominant technique with good results and low complications. The original description described a 130° chevron cut at the neck of the first metatarsal. Alternatively, a transverse or linear cut of the metaphysis could be performed. Both osteotomy configurations are accepted methods of performing MIBS, and each has its advantages and disadvantages.

The chevron osteotomy MIBS is an inherently stabile technique due to the "V" nature as well as increased bone-on-bone contact, which theoretically promotes a high rate of osteotomy consolidation. The transverse osteotomy MIBS has less surface area for bone healing when compared to the chevron. Additionally, the chevron osteotomy also preserves the metatarsal head plantar vascularization, also decreasing the risk of metatarsal head necrosis.[16,36] The transverse osteotomy has a high anatomic risk of injuring the plantar vascularization of the first metatarsal head.[9] Bone healing studies that directly compare these two osteotomy studies have yet to be performed. However, in a retrospective radiographic review characterizing bone healing in 172 feet, Blitz and colleagues[12] introduced a Transveron™ osteotomy MIBS, though there was not a description of the proprietary osteotomy configuration.

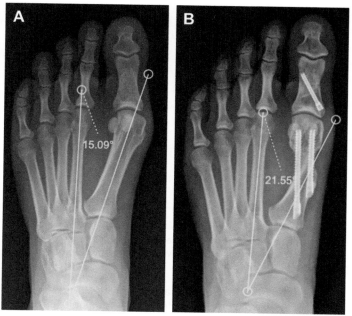

Fig. 3. (A) Preoperative and (B) Postoperative radiograph showing an increased varus displacement of the proximal fragment of the first metatarsal osteotomy.

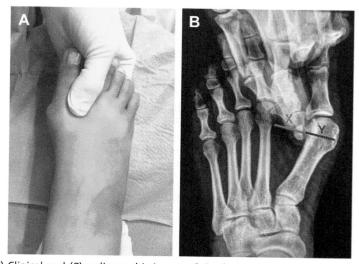

Fig. 4. (A) Clinical and (B) radiographic image of the first ray squeeze test. Observe that a 100% lateral displacement of the metatarsal head covers the first intermetatarsal space. The first metatarsal head size (*green line*; Y) is equal to the intermetatarsal space (*red line*; X).

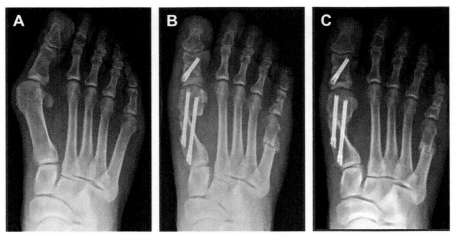

Fig. 5. Radiographic series of a 64 year old male who underwent a transverse osteotomy MIBS. Preoperative (*A*), 06 weeks postoperative and (*B*) and 12 weeks postoperative (*C*) showing a good bone healing.

The 3 dimensional correction can also be achieved with MIBS based on the osteotomy configuration. The "V" cut when translated makes rotation of the metatarsal head difficult, particularly with translations less than 100%. The transverse osteotomy, however, has the ability to correct all severities of coronal/sagittal plane deformity and rotational deformities of the metatarsal articulation regardless of the amount of translation.[6] While the transverse cut allows more rotational correction, it is an inherently unstable osteotomy configuration. The literature on biomechanical studies and clinical trials comparing the 2 osteotomy shapes are still lacking. There is only one biomechanical study carried out in cadavers which compared the transverse and chevron osteotomy in MIBS.[16] Eighteen cadaveric specimens were randomized for both types of osteotomies and submitted to a biomechanical analysis. They demonstrated no significant differences in the load to failure, yield load, and stiffness between chevron and transverse MIBS osteotomy techniques in a cadaveric cantilever bending model.

The authors of the present article believe there is a tendency to use transverse osteotomy (**Fig. 5**). The nature of the transverse cut is maintenance of the Cortical Purchase Zone (CPZ) of the lateral first metatarsal shaft, a necessary portion of the bone require for a stabile fixation construct[6,9,11–13,16] (**Fig. 6**). When a chevron osteotomy is performed its important not to make the "V" cut angle more acute as this could increase the risk of fracture (ie, metatarsal explosion) at the CPZ.[11,13,16,36] Independently of the type of cut, we believe providing a stable rigid fixation construct is necessary, and currently perform this with 2 metatarsal screws as described by Redfern and Vernois.[30]

CONTROVERSY 6: ONE VERSUS TWO METATARSAL SCREW FIXATION

The original Redfern-Vernois chevron-MIBS calls for two compressive metatarsal screws for fixation. With large metatarsal head translations coupled with early weightbearing, rigid and stable fixation has been attributed to its success. Two points of fixation seem to satisfy classic osteotomy/fracture/fusion fixation guidelines providing stability and anti-rotation. A two screw fixation is currently the most utilized and studied fixation construct for MIBS. However, implant-related complications/issues (ie, screw head soft tissue irritation, hardware migration) have necessitating additional procedures.[4,5]

A   B

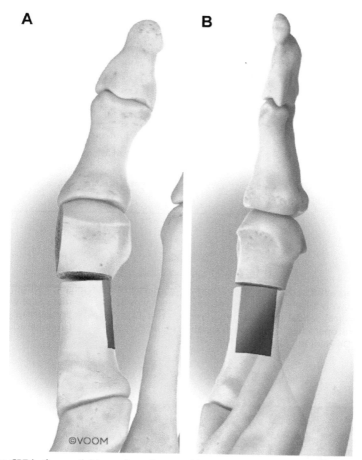

©VOOM

Fig. 6. The CPZ is the available region of cortical bone of the lateral metatarsal shaft (proximal to the osteotomy) where the minimally invasive screw(s) exit. Top-down view (*A*) and view of the lateral first metatarsal (*B*). A transverse osteotomy maximizes the proximal bony real estate adjacent to the osteotomy. (*From:* Reprinted from: Blitz NM, Grecea B, Wong DT, Baskin ES. Defining the Cortical Purchase Zone in New Minimally Invasive Bunion Surgery. A Retrospective Study of 638 Cases. *J Min Invasive Bunion Surg.* 2024;1:92777. doi:10.62485/001c.92777. From: Voom Medical Devices, Inc.)

Single metatarsal screw fixation has also been suggested as an adequate form of MIBS fixation. The largest single metatarsal screw utilization study was performed by Blitz et al (11) when defining the CPZ by measuring the distance from the osteotomy to the where the proximal screw perforates the lateral cortex (a distance defined as the cortical runway). Of the 638 feet in the study, 526 feet (82.4%) has a single metatarsal MI screw. This study involved a single surgeon's first and consecutive cases from January 2018 to November 2022. A single screw construct achieved a mean longer cortical runway when compared to a two screw construct, and was statistically significant. It is inferred that a lengthier cortical runway results in a more stable construct as there is more cortical bone between the screw and osteotomy. They advocate that the ideal fixation construct (in absence of bone brittleness) is for the use of a single

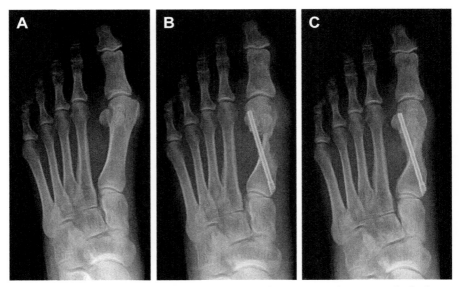

Fig. 7. Radiographic series of a 28 year old woman after MIBS involving a single dual-zone screw paired with a Transveron™ osteotomy. Patient was permitted immediate weightbearing in a surgical sandal after surgery. Preoperative (*A*), 2 weeks postoperative (*B*), and 12 weeks postoperative (*C*) demonstrate the robust first metatarsal regeneration. (*Image courtesy* of Dr. Neal Blitz.)

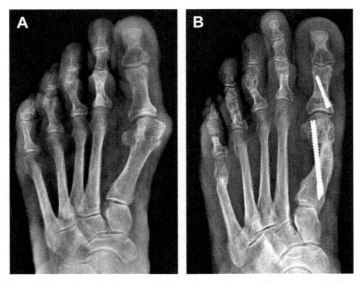

Fig. 8. Radiographic series of a 79 year old female patient with osteoporotic bone who underwent a transverse osteotomy MIBS using a single screw. The authors believe single screw fixation might be particularly advantageous with poor bone quality (combined with a period of nonweightbearing). Preoperative (*A*) and 12 weeks postoperative (*B*).

metatarsal screw originating in the proximal medial first metatarsal base and centered within the metatarsal canal with a lengthy cortical runway.

In 2022, Harrasser and colleagues[37] performed the first comparative study in 50 total patients (33 feet with 2 screws, and 22 feet with 1 screw) with both groups having similar outcomes; however, 32% of patients were dissatisfied with two metatarsal fixation compared to 3% with the single screw. In 2023, Li and colleagues also performed a comparative study in 103 patients in mild-to-moderate HV treated with chevron-MIBS with at least 12 months of follow-up. Both groups (51 patients with single screw fixation and 52 patients with dual screw fixation) had similar outcomes and results.[38] The single metatarsal screw group demonstrated statistically significant lower operative time and less intraoperative fluoroscopy use. There was no nonunion complication in either group. Prominent hardware requiring screw removal was performing 1.9% of the two metatarsal screw and no hardware removal of the single screw group. However, this study involved mild/moderate HV (IM <16°) and its unclear based on this study how single screw outcomes would be for larger bunions.

A large retrospective MIBS study (247 feet) by Mikhail and colleagues mentions use of a single metatarsal screw fixation construct within their cohort; however, they did not mention the frequency of one construct over another.[39] The authors attributed a single metatarsal screw technique to 2.6% of the bone-healing-related complications without any specific construct detail on these particular cases. In 2024, Blitz and colleagues specifically studied bone-healing patterns after MIBS in 172 feet (86% single screw, 14% two screw).[12] They defined the triangular area available for osseus healing as the regeneration triangle, and identified 3 distinct patterns of healing (a term described as FMR). While the study only looked at healed cases, 84% of the single screw fixation feet demonstrated healing lateral to the single screw, and the remaining 16% had primarily medial osseous integration.

The ideal MIBS fixation construct has yet to be determined by clinical studies. Single metatarsal screw fixation shows merit and promise. Recently, an innovative single metatarsal fixation solution was introduced (Revcon™ Anchor Screw—made commercially available by Voom Medical Devices Inc, New York, NY) that has a novel dual-zone pitched shaft to capture the cortical and cancellous aspects of the lateral metatarsal shaft and metatarsal head, respectively (**Fig. 7**). Single metatarsal screw fixation has been advocated by Blitz et al (since 2018), and has further expanded the MIBS generation to fifth and sixth generation to incorporate this construct.[11] In order to make a single screw construct feasible, Blitz recommends pairing it with a stabilizing osteotomy.[40,41] A fifth generation MIBS involves a chevron osteotomy paired with a single compressive or non-compressive MI screw. A sixth generation MIBS involves a new Transveron™ osteotomy (a mix between a chevron and transverse osteotomy) paired with a single dual-zone neutral pitched MI screw.

Future comparative clinical and biomechanical studies are the next logical steps that also evaluate the stability to large/severe metatarsal head displacements. In addition, biomechanical studies would be fundamental to substantiate any overlaps in the types of metatarsal fixation. Osteoporotic poor-quality bone is another variable where single screw fixation might be more advantageous, though the authors propose a minimum of 2 weeks non-weightbearing (**Fig. 8**). The authors, otherwise, currently prefer the use of two metatarsal fixation for MIBS.

SUMMARY

MIBS has evolved in recent years and becoming increasingly popular. While MIBS has become a safe and reliable method to treat HV, there are still controversial and unanswered questions. Future studies will emerge that respond, and resolve, many of the current controversies presented here. The authors believe that MIBS will soon be recognized as the gold standard.

CLINICS CARE POINTS

- It is expected that MIS will become the primary approach for HV, as it has advanced both technically and scientifically.
- It is possible to correct and control the HV rotation parameters. Therefore, it is unclear whether the rotational assessment is indispensable to achieving great results.
- There are a variety of MIS techniques to treat HV. Among them, we have fixed and unfixed techniques, each with its advantages and disadvantages.
- There is a tendency to use the transverse cut in the MIS distal osteotomy since it preserves the medial and lateral cortex and facilitates rotational correction.
- The first ray hipermobility remains as a controversial topic in HV. The MIBS mechanism of first-ray stabilization needs validation with more biomechanical and clinical studies with long-term follow up.
- There is a lack in biomechanical analysis of MIBS fixation. The authors believe that the original MIBS fastening with 2 screws remains the safest and most effective approach.

DISCLOSURE

The authors declare no potential conflicts of interest with respect to the research, authorship, and/or publication of this article. ICMJE forms for all authors are available online. *Financial*: All authors certify that they have no affiliations with or involvement in any organization or entity with any financial interest or non-financial interest in the subject matter or materials discussed in this study. *Consent to publish*: The authors affirm that human research participants provided informed consent to publish the images in figures. The participant has consented to the submission of this case series to the journal.

REFERENCES

1. Ji L, Wang K, Ding S, et al. Minimally invasive vs. open surgery for hallux valgus: a meta-analysis. Front Surg 2022;9:843410.
2. Gonzalez T, Encinas R, Johns W, et al. Minimally invasive surgery using a shannon burr for the treatment of hallux valgus deformity: a systematic review. Foot Ankle Orthop 2023;8(1). 24730114221151069.
3. Zaveri A, Katmeh R, Patel S, et al. The use of intramedullary devices for fixation of metatarsal osteotomies in hallux valgus surgery - a systematic review. Foot Ankle Surg 2022;28(4):483–91.
4. de Carvalho KAM, Baptista AD, de Cesar Netto C, et al. Minimally invasive chevron-Akin for correction of moderate and severe hallux valgus deformities: clinical and radiologic outcomes with a minimum 2-year follow-up. Foot Ankle Int 2022;43(10):1317–30.
5. Nunes GA, de Carvalho KAM, Ferreira GF, et al. Minimally invasive chevron akin (MICA) osteotomy for severe hallux valgus. Arch Orthop Trauma Surg 2023;143(9):5507–14.

6. Lewis TL, Lau B, Alkhalfan Y, et al. Fourth-generation minimally invasive hallux valgus surgery with metaphy- seal extra-articular transverse and akin osteotomy (META): 12 month clinical and radiologic results. Foot Ankle Int 2023; 44(3):178–91.

7. Nunes GA, Ferreira GF, Baumfeld T, et al. Minimally invasive chevron akin: locking the metatarsal-cuneiform joint. Foot Ankle Spec 2022.

8. Lewis TL, Ferreira GF, Nunes GA, et al. Impact of sesamoid coverage on clinical foot function following fourth-generation percutaneous hallux valgus surgery. Foot Ankle Orthop 2024;9(1). 24730114241230560.

9. Nunes GA, Baumfeld T. Third generation rotational percutaneous osteotomy to hallux valgus. Tech Foot Ankle Surg 2023;22(2):65–71.

10. Ferreira GF, Nunes GA, Dorado DS, et al. Correction of first metatarsal pronation in metaphyseal extra-articular transverse osteotomy for hallux valgus correction. Foot Ankle Orthop 2023;8(3). 24730114231198527.

11. Blitz NM, Grecea B, Wong DT, et al. Defining the cortical purchase zone in new minimally invasive bunion surgery. a retrospective study of 638 cases. J Min Invasive Bunion Surg. 2024;1:92777.

12. Blitz NM, Wong DT, Grecea B, et al. Characterization of first metatarsal regeneration after new modern minimally invasive bunion surgery. a retrospective radiographic review of 172 cases. J Min Invasive Bunion Surg. 2024;1.

13. Blitz NM, Wong DT, Baskin ES. Patterns of metatarsal explosion after new modern minimally invasive bunion surgery. a retrospective review and case series of 16 feet. J Min Invasive Bunion Surg. 2024;1:92774.

14. Alimy AR, Polzer H, Ocokoljic A, et al. Does minimally invasive surgery provide better clinical or radiographic outcomes than open surgery in the treatment of hallux valgus deformity? a systematic review and meta-analysis. Clin Orthop Relat Res 2023;481(6):1143–55.

15. Yoon YK, Tang ZH, Shim DW, et al. Minimally invasive transverse distal metatarsal osteotomy (mito) for hallux valgus correction: early outcomes of mild to moderate vs severe deformities. Foot Ankle Int 2023;44(10):992–1002.

16. Aiyer A, Massel DH, Siddiqui N, et al. Biomechanical comparison of 2 common techniques of minimally invasive hallux valgus correction. Foot Ankle Int 2021; 42(3):373–80.

17. Biz C, Fosser M, Dalmau-Pastor M, et al. Functional and radiographic outcomes of hallux valgus correction by mini-invasive surgery with Reverdin-Isham and Akin percutaneous osteotomies: a longitudinal prospective study with a 48-month follow-up. J Orthop Surg Res 2016;11(1):157.

18. Bauer T, de Lavigne C, Biau D, et al. Percutaneous hallux valgus surgery: a prospective multicenter study of 189 cases. Orthop Clin North Am 2009;40(4):505–ix.

19. Molloy A, Widnall J. Scarf osteotomy. Foot Ankle Clin 2014;19(2):165–80.

20. Prado M, Baumfeld T, Nery C, et al. Rotational biplanar Chevron osteotomy. Foot Ankle Surg 2020;26(4):473–6.

21. Song JH, Kang C, Hwang DS, et al. Comparison of radiographic and clinical results after extended distal chevron osteotomy with distal soft tissue release with moderate versus severe hallux valgus. Foot Ankle Int 2019;40(3):297–306.

22. Shibuya N, Kyprios EM, Panchani PN, et al. Factors associated with early loss of hallux valgus correction. J Foot Ankle Surg 2018;57:236–240.4.

23. Jeuken RM, Schotanus MG, Kort NP, et al. Long-term follow-up of a randomized controlled trial comparing Scarf to Chevron osteotomy hallux valgus correction. Foot Ankle Int 2016;37:687–695.5.

24. Bock P, Kluger R, Kristen KH, et al. The Scarf osteotomy with minimally invasive lateral release for the treatment of hallux valgus deformity: intermediate and long-term results. J Bone Joint Surg Am. 2015;97:1238–45.
25. Wagner E, Ortiz C, Gould JS, et al. Proximal oblique sliding closing wedge osteotomy for hallux valgus. Foot Ankle Int 2013;34:1493–1500.9.
26. Yasuda T, Okuda R, Jotoku T, et al. Proximal supination osteotomy of the first metatarsal for hallux valgus. Foot Ankle Int 2015;36:696–704.10.
27. Klemola T, Leppilahti J, Kalinainen S, et al. First tarsometatarsal joint derotational arthrodesis–a new operative technique for flexible hallux valgus without touching the first metatarsophalangeal joint. J Foot Ankle Surg 2014;53:22–8.
28. Kim Y, Kim JS, Young KW, et al. A new measure of tibial sesamoid position in hallux valgus in relation to the coronal rotation of the first metatarsal in CT scans. Foot Ankle Int 2015;36:944–52.
29. Steadman J, Siebert M, Saltzman CL. Sesamoid view x-ray vs weightbearing computed tomography in the measurement of metatarsal pronation angle. Foot Ankle Orthop 2022;7(4). 2473011421S00955.
30. Vernois J, Redfern DJ. Percutaneous surgery for severe hallux valgus. Foot Ankle Clin 2016;21(3):479–93.
31. Kaufmann G, Weiskopf D, Liebensteiner M, et al. Midterm results following minimally invasive distal chevron osteotomy: comparison with the minimally invasive reverdin-isham osteotomy by means of meta-analysis. In Vivo 2021;35(4):2187–96.
32. Biz C, Maso G, Malgarini E, et al. Hypermobility of the first ray: the cinderella of the measurements conventionally assessed for correction of hallux valgus. Acta Biomed 2020;91(4-S):47–59.
33. Roukis TS, Landsman AS. Hypermobility of the first ray: a critical review of the literature. J Foot Ankle Surg 2003;42(6):377–90.
34. Rush SM, Christensen JC, Johnson CH. Biomechanics of the first ray. Part II: metatarsus primus varus as a cause of hypermobility. A three-dimensional kinematic analysis in a cadaver model. J Foot Ankle Surg 2000;39(2):68–77.
35. Cody EA, Caolo K, Ellis SJ, et al. Early radiographic outcomes of minimally invasive chevron bunionectomy compared to the modified lapidus procedure. Foot Ankle Orthop 2022;7(3). 24730114221112103.
36. Lam P, Lee M, Xing J, et al. Percutaneous surgery for mild to moderate hallux valgus. Foot Ankle Clin 2016;21(3):459–77.
37. Harrasser N, Hinterwimmer F, Baumbach SF, et al. The distal metatarsal screw is not always necessary in third-generation MICA: a case–control study. Arch Orthop Trauma Surg 2022;143(8):4633–9.
38. Li X, Zhang J, Fu S, et al. First metatarsal single-screw minimally invasive chevron-akin osteotomy: a cost effective and clinically reliable technique. Front Surg 2023;9:1047168.
39. Mikhail CM, Markowitz J, Di Lenarda L, et al. Clinical and radiographic outcomes of percutaneous chevron-akin osteotomies for the correction of Hallux Valgus deformity. Foot Ankle Int 2021;43(1):32–41.
40. Voom Medical Devices, Co. Revcon minimally invasive screw system surgical technique. Available at: https://www.voommedicaldevices.com/files/2023_Voom_OpTech_Complete_Digital_01.pdf.
41. Blitz NM. New minimally invasive bunion surgery: the End-all Be-all bunion repair? Clin Podiatr Med Surg 2025;42(1):10–31.

Where Minimal Incision Surgery Can Have Maximum Results with Charcot Reconstruction

Matthew Greenblatt, DPM, AACFAS[a], Sara Mateen, DPM, AACFAS[b],
Noman A. Siddiqui, DPM, MHA, FACFAS[a,c],*

KEYWORDS

- Minimally invasive surgery • Charcot deformity correction • Hexapod
- External fixation • Beaming

KEY POINTS

- Comprehend surgical and medical management of Charcot reconstruction as it pertains to the midfoot, hindfoot, and ankle.
- Application of minimally invasive techniques and its evolution toward Charcot reconstruction.
- Application of static and gradual techniques for deformity correction in Charcot patients with case example of midfoot, hindfoot, and ankle deformity.

INTRODUCTION

Charcot neuroarthropathy (CN) poses a therapeutic and management challenge to patients and physicians alike. Characterized by progressive osseous and soft tissue degeneration and remodeling, often compounded by ulceration sequelae, CN remains a limb-threatening deformity. Originally described by Jean-Martin Charcot as a unique joint deterioration pattern among patients with myelopathy secondary to syphilis, the condition presents in association with a spectrum of diagnoses.[1-3] Despite a thorough understanding of CN incidence in conditions from alcoholism to diabetes, the contributing pathophysiology remains debated. The 2 most common explanations include the "neurovascular" and "neurotraumatic" theories.[1-3]

The neurovascular theory postulates that the "trophic" or vasomotor nerve centers disrupt bone and joint nutrition as well as introduce an autonomic component that

[a] International Center of Limb Lengthening, Rubin Institute of Advanced Orthopedics, 2401 West Belvedere Avenue, Baltimore, MD 21215, USA; [b] Hackensack Meridian Health, Division of Orthopedic Surgery, 20 Prospect Avenue, Hackensack, NJ 07601, USA; [c] Division Of Podiatric Surgery, Sinai Hospital, Baltimore, MD, USA
* Corresponding author.
E-mail address: nsiddiqu@lifebridgehealth.org

Clin Podiatr Med Surg 42 (2025) 167–176
https://doi.org/10.1016/j.cpm.2024.06.002
0891-8422/25/© 2024 Elsevier Inc. All rights are reserved, including those for text and data mining, AI training, and similar technologies.

dysregulates smooth muscle tone. This is speculated to have a deleterious effect on the arterial wall, leading to a failure in vasoregulation, increased blood flow to the bone, and subsequent overactive osteoclastic formation, resulting in accelerated bone resorption.[4] The neurotraumatic theory holds simply that an insensate foot may be prone to repetitive unrecognized trauma due to loss of proprioception, causing chronic abnormal joint loading and biomechanical breakdown.[2]

The goal of CN management is to establish a stable braceable plantigrade foot. In the absence of infection or ulceration, accommodative footwear with custom insoles and a rigid shank can be helpful. A Charcot restraint orthotic walker or ankle foot orthosis are also useful options. These conservative measures may support a reduced inflammatory response, potentially delaying deformity progression.[5-8] In addition, pharmacologic agents such as antiosteoporotic drugs and bisphosphonates may offer some added benefit, though they may not be viable in the long term.[9]

While conservative treatment may be useful in some patients, prolonged immobilization may be cumbersome, particularly in the elderly population. Greater than 18 months of immobilization can carry an amputation rate of up to 2.7% and a 49% risk of recurrent ulcerations.[10] In addition to the risks inherent to prolonged immobilization, conservative treatment is not indicated in those with a nonplantigrade foot, with or without ulceration. Surgical intervention may range from soft tissue release, wound debridement and exostectomy, to full reconstruction with deformity correction via internal and/or external fixation.[7-11]

This article will provide a comprehensive review of minimally invasive surgery (MIS) management techniques for Charcot reconstruction and acute versus gradual deformity correction of the midfoot, hindfoot, and ankle.

MINIMALLY INVASIVE TECHNIQUES FOR CHARCOT RECONSTRUCTION

MIS has evolved within foot and ankle surgery, particularly with respect to bunion surgery.[12-17] Bosch and colleagues provided some of the earliest publications, describing MIS hallux valgus correction with a 1 cm incision over the first metatarsal head and neck. Their technique involved fixation with a 2 mm Steinman pin, resulting in excellent radiographic outcomes with up to 95% patient satisfaction.[18,19] Giannini and Isham[20,21] corroborated these findings, presenting their success with minimally invasive hallux valgus correction. Siddiqui and colleagues have also reported the efficacy of minimally invasive bunion surgery, with over 300 procedures performed. With the advent of these improved techniques and technology, outcomes have been overall more favorable.[22-24]

Beyond hallux valgus surgery, minimally invasive techniques have been popularized in hammertoe correction, exostectomies, calcaneal osteotomies, trauma reconstruction, and Charcot reconstruction.[14-17,25-27] In Charcot reconstruction with a minimally invasive approach, important principles remain consistent with traditional Association of Osteosynthesis/Arbeitsgemeinschaft für Osteosynthesefragen (AO) surgical guidelines including minimal soft tissue disruption, preserved vascularity, and anatomic reduction, which in turn facilitates mechanical realignment, stability maintenance, and early mobilization.[26,27] Neuropathic MIS "NEMISIS" has been described specifically with intramedullary column beaming. This is an important concept in CN, as patients are at an increased risk of wound complications, hardware failure, and postoperative infection.[27]

Minimally invasive techniques for midfoot Charcot reconstruction are built around the guiding principles of adjacent joint arthrodesis, stable intraosseous fixation, anatomic realignment, preservation of foot length, and awareness of possible external fixation needs.[28] With the advancement of surgical techniques, technology, and instrumentation,

MIS has given surgeons the means to optimize outcomes while minimizing the surgical biologic footprint. These benefits have been well reported in the literature, such as less soft tissue disruption, preservation of periosteal blood supply, minimized postoperative pain, and lower incidence of wound-related complications.[11,29–34]

MIDFOOT CHARCOT RECONSTRUCTION

The surgical principles of neuroarthropathy joint reconstruction have centered often on bony realignment with minimal discussion on the soft tissue contractures that, perhaps, exacerbate the bone malalignment. The tendo Achilles is routinely implicated as a major deforming force, and this has been documented.[26] However, the other deforming forces are often overlooked, and a global consideration to the soft tissue must be included when correcting the collapse.

The senior author has found appropriate lengthening of tendons and capsule is necessary to achieve a successful outcome. The senior author's (NAS) goal in MIS midfoot Charcot reconstruction is to balance the frontal plane deforming forces by neutralizing the soft tissue imbalance that can occur from pedal collapse. An important biomechanical concept is to recognize that the ground reactive forces about the subtalar and ankle joint do not disappear when pedal neuroarthropathy is present. The extrinsic musculature responsible for stabilizing and assisting in gait from heel strike to toe off continue to fire whenever gait is initiated. However, the insensate foot combined with joint destruction will convert normal gait pattern events into deforming forces that worsen the collapse commonly seen through the midfoot. Therefore, it is equally important to address the soft tissue deforming forces simultaneously with the re-establishment of bony stability. The goal at the end of the soft tissue release and re-establishing bony alignment is to negate the frontal plane influence on the insensate foot and ankle while maintaining adequate strength from the anterior compartment for dorsiflexion and supporting plantarflexion with the assistance of the deep flexors excluding the posterior tibial tendon and Achilles tendon.

Sagittal Plane Relaxation: Posterior Muscle Group Lengthening

The procedure generally begins with posterior muscular group lengthening. While the gastrocnemius recession reduces the risk of overlengthening and calcaneal gait, patients with midfoot Charcot can often have significant posterior muscular and capsular contractures that are not adequately reduced with a traditional gastrocnemius recession. We typically perform either a modified Vulpius or Z-lengthening of the tendo Achilles. In severe contractures, an Achilles lengthening through a 3 cm lateral incision can be necessary when performing hindfoot/ankle arthrodesis. This is performed just proximal to the combined gastrocnemius and soleus tendon complex. The aponeurosis of the gastrocnemius and soleus muscle is safe location to perform this maneuver. The lengthening significantly attenuates the plantarflexory-deforming cantilever midfoot forces imparted by the combination of the hindfoot equinus contracture and ground reactive forces.

Frontal/Transverse Plane Stabilization: Peroneal and Posterior Tibial Tendon Tenotomy

The most common location for Charcot breakdown is the tarsometatarsal joints, which can lead to rocker bottom deformity with plantar, medial, or lateral osseous prominences, with or without valgus drift of the forefoot. There are soft tissue opposing forces from the extrinsic dorsiflexors and extensors with a contracted Achilles tendon that exacerbate midfoot dislocation, or "bayonetting" of the forefoot upon the hindfoot

(**Fig. 1**). In turn, this typically follows a dorsolateral pattern due to the longitudinal pull of the anterior tibial tendon and posterior muscle groups. The peroneal tendons will further lock the forefoot on the midfoot/hindfoot due to the role of the peroneal brevis and longus tendons once the cuneiforms and cuboid collapse occurs. This combined with the antagonistic roles of the posterior tibial and anterior tibial tendons further worsen the midfoot locking seen with bayonet deformities. To minimize the role of these deforming forces, we perform a release of the peroneus longus and brevis tendons.

The surgical technique to release the peroneal tendons is done through a small linear incision at the lateral fibular border, where the tendons are visualized at transected with a 15 blade. After identifying the lateral fibular border, a 1.5 cm longitudinal incision is made. In the presence of lateral ankle instability, we preserve the peroneus brevis tendon, which can be utilized in a nonanatomic repair to lateral ankle stabilization procedure.

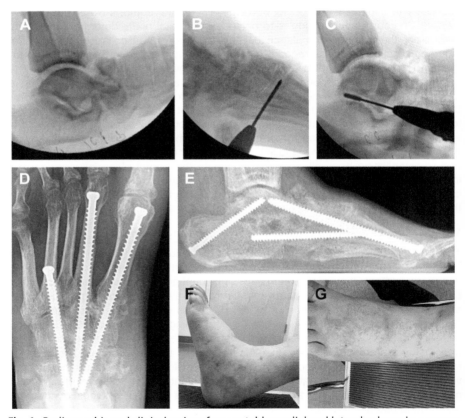

Fig. 1. Radiographic and clinical series of an unstable medial and lateral column in a neuropathic patient with a history of recurrent chronic midfoot ulceration. (*A*) Tarsal collapse evident on fluoroscan. (*B*) Intraoperative fluoroscopic image of percutaneous midfoot fusion preparation with Shannon bur. (*C*) Subtalar fusion joint preparation via percutaneous approach under fluoroscopy using a Wedge bur. (*D, E*) Radiographs 1 year after arthrodesis of the midfoot and subtalar joint resulting in realigned stable foot. (*F, G*) Corresponding clinical images at 1 year with supple soft tissue envelope with healed percutaneous incisions. (With permission from Dr. Noman A. Siddiqui, D.P.M., Sinai Hospital of Baltimore and the Rubin Institute for Advanced Orthopedics.)

Posterior Tibial Tendon Tenotomy

After the peroneal tendons are released, the posterior tibial tendon is then released at the navicular tuberosity via a 1 cm incision. The dual benefit of incisional placement at this level is to further serve as portals for placement of the minimally invasive surgical burs that will be utilized for osteotomy/joint prep. Following the release of these soft tissue contractures, mobility of the foot in multiple planes is achieved allowing for appropriate reduction of the triplanar deformity. If needed, the incision is extended proximally or distally to release the capsular contraction of the midfoot. However, this maneuver may not be necessary if gradual correction with an external fixator is planned.

Minimally Invasive Midfoot Osteotomy

Attention is then directed to the midfoot. Under fluoroscopic guidance, 1.8 mm Ilizarov wires are inserted through incisions at the medial aspect of the navicular and the lateral aspect of the cuboid to map out the trajectory of the osteotomy site. Once the proper trajectory of wires is configured, a 15 blade is used to make a percutaneous incision at the wire level. A bur is then inserted to osteotomized through the naviculo-cuneiform joint and cuboid or calcaneocuboid joint. In some cases, the navicular has dislocated or developed multisegmented dissolution. In such scenarios, the bur will morselize the remaining navicular segments. A high torque and low-speed bur with continuous irrigation are utilized to reduce the risk of thermal necrosis. This will result in desirable segmental shortening of the osseous architecture, without the need for large wedge resection (**Fig. 2**). This facilitates positioning the foot optimally for either acute or gradual correction. Confirmation of complete osteotomy is noted under fluoroscopy with mobility of the forefoot upon the hindfoot.

Joint Preparation

Joint preparation follows the same principles of the minimally invasive midfoot osteotomy. Under fluoroscopic guidance, a percutaneous incision is made near every joint that can be accessed for prep. In general, plantar medial and dorsal lateral incisions are employed over the Lisfranc/tarsometatarsal level, naviculocuneiform level, talonavicular level, and sinus tarsi. These 5 to 8 mm incisions serve as entry portals for the bur to prep the joints to achieve formal arthrodesis as a general principle. Under fluoroscopic guidance, the bur is inserted at the joint and, once confirmed, cartilage is denuded from the articular surface. Fenestration of the subchondral plate can be performed to increase osseous perfusion for further consolidation. Liberal use of fluoroscopy is necessary to ensure loss of subchondral bone and cartilage space. Small joint arthroscopy can be employed.

Midfoot Reduction with Application of Multiplanar External Fixation

After the soft tissue releases, midfoot osteotomy, and joint preparation are performed, internal or external fixation is then employed. This is considered "stage 1" of the midfoot Charcot reconstruction. When there is significant deformity present, gradual correction with hexapod external fixation utilizing a butt frame is executed. Manual correction is performed intraoperatively with residual correction performed gradually. This is an important concept, as this minimally invasive approach to midfoot Charcot revolves around obtaining axial distraction and translational relative realignment to obtain a stable tripod. Given the minimal incisions needed for soft tissue release, the hexapod is activated over a short 5 to 7 day latency period. Patients are educated

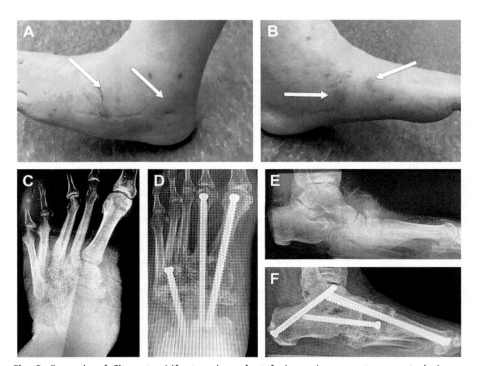

Fig. 2. Example of Charcot midfoot and rearfoot fusion using percutaneous techniques. (*A, B*) Incision portal locations (*white arrows*) for joint preparation and arthrodesis. (*C, D*) Preoperative radiographs of unstable collapsed Charcot midfoot deformity with fragmentation. (*E, F*) Postoperative radiographs at 2 years after successful arthrodesis of midfoot and rearfoot joints resulting in a plantargrade foot. (With permission from Dr. Noman A. Siddiqui, D.P.M., Sinai Hospital of Baltimore and the Rubin Institute for Advanced Orthopedics.)

postoperatively about how to perform the turns and properly maintain external fixation.

MIDFOOT CHARCOT RECONSTRUCTION WITH BEAMING

"Stage 2" involves either converting the gradual correction device into a rigid static device or placing rigid internal fixations. Selection of the method is based on the presence of any open wounds. If open wounds are present, the gradual device will be converted into a rigid static fixator to allow load transfer. If no wounds are present and there are no active areas of concern for osteomyelitis, internal fixation is placed previously described by the senior author (NAS).[26] This will consist of beaming the medial and the lateral columns, as well as performing a subtalar joint arthrodesis.[35] Modifying the concepts of superconstructs has been helpful to reinforce principles of correction:

1. Extension of the arthrodesis beyond the zone of injury to maximize contact between the fixation and solid bone,
2. Distraction with gradual correction with selective soft tissue release allowing for stronger reconstruction without soft tissue tension, and
3. Utilization of rigid fixation without compromising soft tissue integrity while promoting biomechanical stability.

The intramedullary screw fixation is a key component. It serves to limit soft tissue dissection and confers biomechanical stability by minimizing cantilever-bending forces that could compromise the plantar aspect of the reconstruction. Our protocol is to routinely fuse the subtalar joint for the purpose of limiting frontal plane motion while the medial and lateral column beams limit transverse and sagittal plane motion, thus, enhancing stability and delaying further Charcot collapse.[35]

Many patients will complete their surgical treatment at stage 2, but if a static external fixator remains in place, a "stage 3" comprising of external fixation removal and subsequent casting may be necessary. If a wound or other concern for infection is present, internal fixation is not performed and external fixation remains in place while the patient is treated with local wound care and antibiotics. Stage 3 can recommence with device removal once negative cultures are obtained and the soft tissue envelope is fully healed.

HINDFOOT AND ANKLE CHARCOT RECONSTRUCTION
Charcot Reconstruction Without Talectomy

In hindfoot Charcot, tibiotalocalcaneal arthrodesis is a viable treatment with several methods of fixation. The most utilized option is a retrograde intramedullary nail with locking screw fixation, though large, cannulated screws may be used as well. The joint preparation is minimally invasive, with small medial and lateral ankle arthrotomy incisions overlying the ankle joint. Under fluoroscopy, the bur placement is confirmed for both the medial and lateral ankle joints to ensure proper joint preparation. The ankle joint is prepped utilizing multiple sizes of burs. The entire joint, including the gutters, is denuded of cartilage with exposure of bleeding, cancellous bone. In certain scenarios, the calcaneus needs to be medialized under the hindfoot. If this scenario is present, a medial malleolar osteotomy is performed to align the hindfoot with the tibia. This is checked fluoroscopically with a calcaneal axial view and temporarily pinned in place prior to final fixation. As with midfoot Charcot reconstruction, the subtalar joint is always prepped for fusion. The sinus tarsi is palpated and a 5 mm incision is performed. Under fluoroscopic guidance, the bur is inserted into the subtalar joint and once confirmed, cartilage is denuded of the posterior, middle, and anterior facets. Once all the joints are prepped, proper technique for intramedullary nail fixation is applied. Patients are placed in a below-knee cast postoperatively and instructed to observe 50% weight-bearing.

Charcot Reconstruction with Talectomy and Distal Tibial Lengthening

Hindfoot and ankle Charcot poses a challenge among experienced foot and ankle surgeons, as many patients experience soft tissue deformity and osseous fragmentation with infection. Given the severity of these deformities with resection of nonviable bone, segmental bone loss typically ensues. In the setting of a talectomy, a tibiocalcaneal arthrodesis is performed with distal tibial distraction osteogenesis via external fixation. Siddiqui and colleagues[36,37] reported a 93.3% arthrodesis success rate in 15 patients with a mean time to full consolidation at 9.8 months.

In the presence of a wound with concern for infection, a staged approach is performed, starting with excision of wound and all nonviable bone, hardware removal (if needed), intraoperative cultures, and placement of polymethylmethacrylate spacer and off-loading external fixator (if indicated). This will remain in place for 6 to 8 weeks depending on the duration of the intravenous antibiotics regimen and the ability to obtain clean margins and negative cultures. In the absence of a wound where there remains concern for talar avascular necrosis or infection, the talectomy is performed through a full thickness standard lateral approach via an oblique transverse incision. The peroneal tendons are tenotomized and 3 cm of the distal fibula is resected to access the tibiotalar and tibiocalcaneal joints. Once the compromised talus material is identified, it is removed in segments until its entirety is excised. The articular surfaces of the distal tibia and calcaneus are then removed with a combination of curettes, low speed burs, and osteotomies. These exposed, bleeding surfaces will create a "cup-like" fit and is temporarily fixated in place. Following this, a hexapod external fixator is built utilizing a 2 tibial ring block proximally, 1 tibial ring distal to the osteotomy, and a footplate. The distal tibial/supramalleolar minimally invasive osteotomy is performed approximately 5 cm from the arthrodesis site at the metaphyseal diaphyseal junction, with the goal of 5 to 8 mm acute compression. This is performed through mini-open or percutaneous incisions via a low-speed bur or using a multiple drill-hole technique. Six-axis multiplanar struts allow for distraction osteogenesis, connecting the distal tibial ring from the proximal ring block to the distal tibial ring. Axial lengthening is initiated approximately 14 to 17 days postoperatively, and patients can be 50% weight-bearing with an assistive device. Serial radiographs are assessed during follow-up. Once adequate stability of the regenerate and consolidation of the arthrodesis site are achieved, a permanent retrograde intramedullary nail with locking screw fixation is inserted.

SUMMARY

CN is an unpredictable disease with a progressive pathology that affects quality of life. Proper clinical and radiographic workup is necessary to provide the patient with the optimal level of care for limb preservation. MIS can limit soft tissue disruption, preserve vascularity, obtain anatomic reduction, and promote early mobilization, which provides particularly important benefits in such a complex patient population. The senior author has utilized minimal incision, mini-open, and percutaneous methods to restore the pedal alignment of the foot, ankle, and supramalleolar level with success. The benefit of decreasing the biologic surgical footprint created by these methods is, perhaps, one way to limit the soft tissue challenges that can occur with large open incisions. The authors recommend a comprehensive approach in this patient population and feel minimally invasive methods should be added to the armamentarium of musculoskeletal surgeons managing CN.

CLINICS CARE POINTS

- Minimally invasive reconstruction demonstrates decreased wound complication.
- Superconstructs enhance the stability of the reconstruction.
- Subtalar joint fusion can decrease hindfoot and ankle collapse in neuropathic reconstruction.
- Distraction osteogenesis performed distally can improve arthrodesis rates in neuropathic fusion of the tibio-talocalcaneal complex.

DISCLOSURE

S. Mateen and M. Greenblatt have no financial disclosures or conflicts of interest. N.A. Siddiqui is a consultant for Arthrex. The following organizations supported the institution of M. Greenblatt, S. Mateen, and N.A. Siddiqui: DePuy Synthes, United States,

NuVasive Specialized Orthopedics, United States, Orthofix, United States, OrthoPediatrics, Paragon 28, Pega Medical, Smith & Nephew, United Kingdom, Stryker, United States, Turner Imaging Systems, and WishBone Medical.

REFERENCES

1. Edmonds ME. Progress in care of the diabetic foot. Lancet 1999;354:270–2.
2. Charcot JM. Sur quelques arthropathies qui paraissent dependre d'une lesion du cerveau ou de la moelle epiniere. Arch Des Phys Norm et Pathol 1868;1:161.
3. Harris A, Violand M. Charcot neuropathic osteoarthropathy. In: StatPearls [Internet]. Treasure Island (FL): StatPearls Publishing; 2023.
4. Chisholm KA, Gilchrist JM. The Charcot joint: a modern neurologic perspective. J Clin Neuromuscul Dis 2011;13:1–13.
5. Vopat ML, Nentwig MJ, Chong ACM, et al. Initial diagnosis and management for acute Charcot neuroarthropathy. Kans J Med 2018;11(4):114–9.
6. Blume PA, Sumpio B, Schmidt B, et al. Charcot neuroarthropathy of the foot and ankle: diagnosis and management strategies. Clin Podiatr Med Surg 2014;31(1): 151–72.
7. Parisi MCR, Godoy-Santos AL, Ortiz RT, et al. Radiographic and functional results in the treatment of early stages of Charcot neuroarthropathy with a walker boot and immediate weight bearing. Diabet Foot Ankle 2013;4(1). https://doi.org/10. 3402/dfa.v4i0.22487.
8. Pinzur MS, Lio T, Posner M. Treatment of Eichenholtz stage I Charcot foot arthropathy with a weightbearing total contact cast. Foot Ankle Int 2006;27(5):324–9.
9. Pitocco D, Scavone G, Di Leo M, et al. Charcot neuroarthropathy: from the laboratory to the bedside. Curr Diabetes Rev 2019;16(1):62–72.
10. Saltzman CL, Hagy ML, Zimmerman B, et al. How effective is intensive nonoperative initial treatment of patients with diabetes and Charcot arthropathy of the feet? Clin Orthop Relat Res 2005;435:185–90.
11. LaPorta GA, D'Andelet A. Lengthen, alignment, and beam technique for midfoot Charcot neuroarthropathy. Clin Podiatr Med Surg 2018;35(4):497–507.
12. Mikhail CM, Markowitz J, Di Lenarda L, et al. Clinical and radiographic outcomes of percutaneous chevron-akin osteotomies for the correction of hallux valgus deformity. Foot Ankle Int 2022;43:32–41.
13. Lewis TL, Robinson PW, Ray R, et al. Five-year follow-up of third-generation percutaneous chevron and Akin osteotomies (PECA) for hallux valgus. Foot Ankle Int 2023;44(2):104–17.
14. Kheir E, Borse V, Sharpe J, et al. Medial displacement calcaneal osteotomy using minimally invasive technique. Foot Ankle Int 2015;36(3):248–52.
15. Kendal AR, Khalid A, Ball T, et al. Complications of minimally invasive calcaneal osteotomy versus open osteotomy. Foot Ankle Int 2015;36(6):685–90.
16. Coleman MM, Abousayed MM, Thompson JM, et al. Risk factors for complications associated with minimally invasive medial displacement calcaneal osteotomy. Foot Ankle Int 2021;42(2):121–31.
17. Carranza-Bencano A, Tejero S, del Castillo-Blanco G, et al. Minimal incision surgery for tibiotalocalcaneal arthrodesis. Foot Ankle Int 2014;35(3):272–84.
18. Bocsch P, Markowski H, Rannicher V. Technik und erste ergebnisse der subkutanen distalen metatarsale, I osteotomie. Orthopaedische Praxis 1990;26:51–6.
19. Bocsch P, Wanke S, Legenstein R. Hallux valgus correction by the method of Bocsch: a new technique with a seven-to-ten-year follow-up. Foot Ankle Clin 2000;5(3):485–98.

20. Isham SA. The Reverdin-Isham procedure for the correction of hallux abducto valgus. a distal metatarsal osteotomy procedure. Clin Podiatr Med Surg 1991; 8(1):81–94.
21. Giannini S, Ceccarelli F, Bevoni R, et al. Hallux valgus surgery: the minimally invasive bunion correction (SERI). Tech Foot Ankle Surg 2003;2(1):11–20.
22. Botek G, Figas S, Narra S. Charcot neuroarthropathy advances: understanding pathogenesis and medical and surgical management. Clin Podiatr Med Surg 2019;36(4):663–84.
23. Siddiqui NA, LaPorta GA. Minimally invasive bunion correction. Clin Podiatr Med Surg 2018;35(4):387–402.
24. Siddiqui NA, LaPorta G, Walsh AL, et al. Radiographic outcomes of a percutaneous, reproducible distal metatarsal osteotomy for mild and moderate bunions: a multicenter study. J Foot Ankle Surg 2019;58(6):1215–22.
25. Superconstructs in the treatment of Charcot foot deformity: plantar plating, locked plating, and axial screw fixation. Foot Ankle Clin 2009;14(3):393–407.
26. Siddiqui NA, LaPorta GA. Midfoot charcot reconstruction. Clin Podiatr Med Surg 2018;35(4):509–20.
27. Miller RJ. Neuropathic minimally invasive surgeries (NEMESIS): percutaneous diabetic foot surgery and reconstruction. Foot Ankle Clin 2016;21(3):595–627.
28. Lamm BM, Siddiqui NA, Nair AK, et al. Intramedullary foot fixation for midfoot Charcot neuroarthropathy. J Foot Ankle Surg 2012;51(4):531–6.
29. Manchanda K, Wallace SB, Ahn J, et al. Charcot midfoot reconstruction: does subtalar arthrodesis or medial column fixation improve outcomes? J Foot Ankle Surg 2020;59(6):1219–23.
30. Lee DJ, Schaffer J, Chen T, et al. Internal versus external fixation of charcot midfoot deformity realignment. Orthopedics 2016;39(4):e595–601.
31. DuBois KS, Cates NK, O'Hara NN, et al. Coronal hindfoot alignment in midfoot charcot neuroarthropathy. J Foot Ankle Surg 2022;61(5):1039–45.
32. Kwaadu KY. Charcot reconstruction: understanding and treating the deformed charcot neuropathic arthropathic foot. Clin Podiatr Med Surg 2020;37(2):247–61.
33. Crim BE, Lowery NJ, Wukich DK. Internal fixation techniques for midfoot charcot neuroarthropathy in patients with diabetes. Clin Podiatr Med Surg 2011;28(4): 673–85.
34. Perren SM. The biomechanics and biology of internal fixation using plates and nails. Orthopedics 1989;12(1):21–34.
35. Mateen S, Thomas MA, Jappar A, et al. Progression to hindfoot charcot neuroarthropathy after midfoot charcot correction in patients with and without subtalar joint arthrodesis. J Foot Ankle Surg 2023;62(4):731–6.
36. Millonig KJ, Siddiqui NA. Tibial lengthening and intramedullary nail fixation for hindfoot charcot neuroarthropathy. Clin Podiatr Med Surg 2022;39(4):659–73.
37. Siddiqui NA, Millonig KJ, Mayer BE, et al. Increased arthrodesis rates in charcot neuroarthropathy utilizing distal tibial distraction osteogenesis principles. Foot Ankle Spec 2022;15(4):394–408.